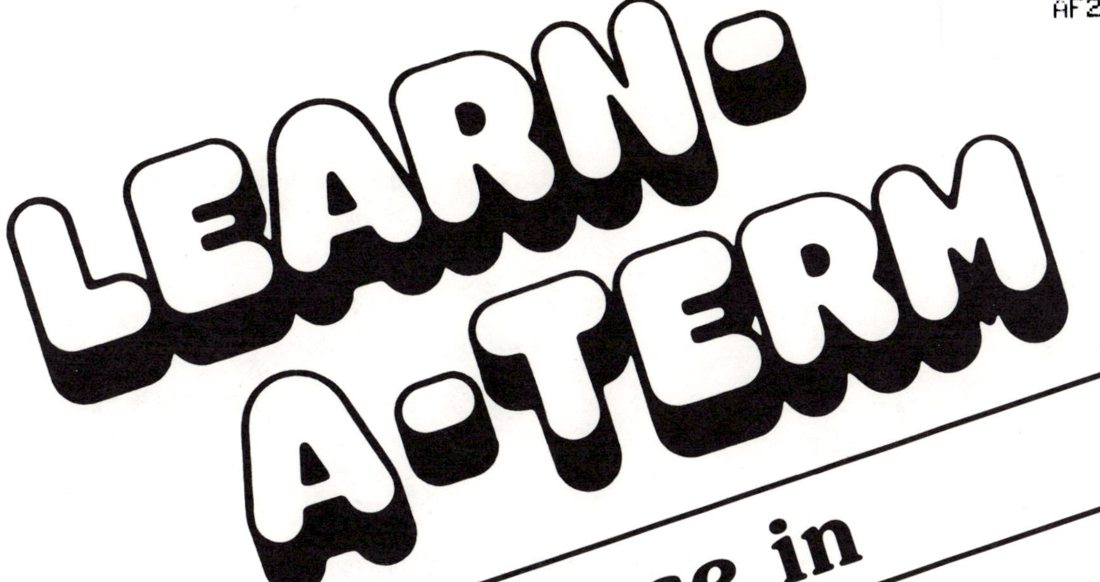

LEARN-A-TERM

A Course in Medical Terminology

**A. Brent Garber
and Leroy Sparks**

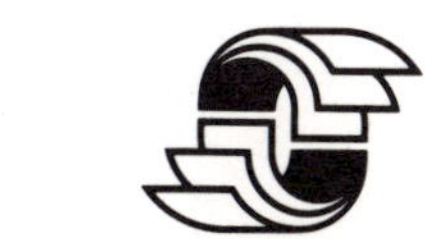

AN ASPEN PUBLICATION®
Aspen Publishers, Inc.
Gaithersburg, Maryland
1977

Library of Congress Cataloging-in-Publication Data

Learn-A-Term: A course in Medical Terminology/
A. Brent Garber and Leroy Sparks

The authors have made every effort to ensure the accuracy of the information herein. However, appropriate information sources should be consulted, especially for new or unfamiliar procedures. It is the responsibility of every practitioner to evaluate the appropriateness of a particular opinion in the context of actual clinical situations and with due consideration to new developments. Authors, editors, and the publisher cannot be held responsible for any typographical or other errors found in this book.

Library of Congress Catalog Card Number: 77-82026
ISBN: 0-912862-48-3

Printed in the United States of America

11 12 13 14 15

Table of Contents

Preface

Several years ago while conducting communications and reading programs for management in large New York hospitals, I met with the then training director of Mt. Sinai Hospital, Paul Cirincioni, who said the real need of the hospital was not in the area of management but with the people who had no medical background and who needed to use medical terms. I agreed that if the training department of Mt. Sinai would supply the terms, we, the Human Research Laboratories, would try to write a program that would teach 200 medical terms in a day.

After many trial classes conducted jointly with Mt. Sinai, *Learn-a-Term* was born. Its success was probably its simplicity, making the boring task of learning medical terms a little bit fun. Since then the program has been well received at major hospitals and has also been taught on the university level at Hostos Community College in New York.

Our intention is to teach you the useful terms quickly and easily and, hopefully, to give you some visual devices to make learning fun.

A. Brent Garber, Ph.D.

Professor Leroy Sparks
Chairman, Radiology Department
Downstate Medical College

July 1977

Introduction

LEARN-A-TERM is a course in medical terminology especially designed to measure and increase your comprehension of many of the words you encounter in the course of your work, but whose meanings and applications may be unclear or unknown to you. The course is in no way a test of your abilities; rather it is meant to be used as a tool to make your job more meaningful and rewarding while at the same time enabling you to improve your own performance.

There is a variety of teaching methods employed in this program. You will take an initial pre-test to determine your current level of comprehension. Once you have isolated those words which are unknown or unclear to you, you will—through a series of matching, fill-in-the-blank, and true and false exercises, combined with crossword puzzles—break these words down into their various parts (prefix, root, suffix). Attached to each of these word parts is a cartoon-style memory device designed to assist you in creating lasting memory associations.

As you go through the exercises, keep referring to the instructions; they will explain what must be done in each case.

Pre-test Instructions

The LEARN-A-TERM pre-test consists of 202 words, each with four possible definitions, only one of which is correct. The object of this pre-test is to determine which of these words you do not know. It is important, therefore, that you select answers only for those words you believe you know. DO NOT GUESS.

You may use the answer sheet provided on page 15.

As you read each word and group of definitions, select the definition you believe to be correct. Enter the corresponding letter in the appropriate blank. For those words you do not know, place an X in the answer space. The example below shows the procedure to be followed.

Pre-test Answer Sheet

1. X	25. 1	49. 2	73. 1	97. X	121. X	145. 2
2. 3	26. X	50. 3	74. X	98. X	122. 4	146. 3
3. 4	27. 3	51. 1	75. X	99. 4	123. X	147. X
4. X	28. X	52. X	76. X	100. 2	124. 1	148. 1

To check your answers, turn to page 151. Place an X over all answers which are incorrect. Be sure to check all 202 answers. Total up all the correct answers and record this number on the answer sheet in the "score" space provided in the lower right hand corner. Then subtract this number from the total 202 index words. You will then have the number of words you have to learn.

Remember that this is not a test of your knowledge or abilities, but simply a first step in teaching you those words which will benefit and enrich your job and your job performance.

Index/Multiple Choice Pre-test

1. C1   **Abdomen** — (1) small intestine; (2) large intestine; (3) cavity containing stomach; (4) cavity containing lungs.

2. C1 D1   **Abdominal** — (1) relating to the solar plexus; (2) relating to the small intestine; (3) relating to the abdominal cavity; (4) stomach operation.

3. C1 D3   **Abdominocentesis** — (1) removal of appendix; (2) removal of blood from abdomen; (3) puncture of large intestine; (4) abdominal puncture to let out air.

4. C2   **Acquired** — (1) developed after birth; (2) contracted; (3) infected; (4) contagious.

5. C3   **Acute** — (1) fatal; (2) rapid course and short duration; (3) sudden; (4) slow process and long duration.

6. A2 D15   **Adenoid** — (1) painful joints; (2) muscle cramp; (3) gland-like; (4) muscle tumor.

7. A2 D17   **Adenoma** — (1) fibrous tissue tumors; (2) glandular tissue tumors; (3) muscle tumor; (4) painful stomach.

8. A3 D24   **Adhesion** — (1) abnormal sticking together; (2) tumor; (3) injury; (4) crack in bone.

9. C4   **Airway** — (1) lungs; (2) nose; (3) mouth; (4) entire breathing passage.

10. C5 C53   **Anaphylactic Shock** — (1) shock occurring after injection of drug because of allergy to drug; (2) shock after accident; (3) shock after severe blood loss; (4) shock after drug overdose.

11. A4 D25   **Anastomosis** — (1) inflammation of the lung; (2) painful stomach; (3) join two parts to make new passageway; (4) overbreathing.

12. A5 D9   **Aneurysm** — (1) injury to head; (2) bruise; (3) shortage of oxygen in blood; (4) ballooning out of blood vessel.

13. A6 D6   **Angiography** — (1) picture of spinal cord; (2) picture of blood vessels; (3) bursting forth of blood; (4) muscle tumor.

14. A6 D26   **Angiospasm** — (1) fast heartbeat; (2) stoppage of heart; (3) blood clot; (4) vessel cramp.

15. A1 D11   **Anomaly** — (1) a sickness; (2) tear in skin; (3) area of diseased tissue; (4) vary from normal.

16. A1 D12   **Anorexia** — (1) fluid in tissue; (2) vague feeling of illness; (3) loss of appetite; (4) cessation of breathing.

17. A1 D13   **Anoxia** — (1) loss of blood; (2) shallow breathing; (3) shortage of oxygen; (4) death by suffocation.

18. C6 **Anus** — (1) sac or bladder with fluid in it; (2) opening at end of digestive tract; (3) sore inside digestive tract; (4) hole in abdominal wall.

19. A1 **Apnea** — (1) overbreathing; (2) temporary stoppage of breathing; (3) sign of disease; (4) fluid in
D21   tissue.

20. C7 **Apoplexy** — (1) heart attack; (2) dizziness; (3) nausea; (4) paralysis and fainting due to stroke.

21. C8 **Appendectomy** — (1) removal of anus; (2) removal of appendix; (3) removal of part of small in-
D4   testine; (4) cutting off of pancreas.

22. C8 **Appendix** — (1) sac producing bile; (2) sac producing red blood cells; (3) sac off large intestine; (4)
sac near liver.

23. A7 **Arthralgia** — (1) inflammation of bone; (2) cracking of bone; (3) painful joints; (4) tendon inflam-
D2   mation.

24. A7 **Arthritis** — (1) inflammation of joints; (2) skin tumor; (3) inflammation of the arm; (4) the small
D10   intestine.

25. C9 **Ascites** — (1) fluid in abdominal cavity; (2) too little oxygen in the blood; (3) inflammation of the
arm; (4) brain covering.

26. A1 **Aseptic** — (1) containing germs; (2) free of pus-producing germs; (3) removal of tumor; (4) not free
C52   of pus-producing germs.

27. A1 **Atrophy** — (1) excessive growth; (2) severe, recurring; (3) mild, not recurring; (4) wasting away of
D28   body parts.

28. C10 **Benign** — (1) severe and growing worse; (2) shifting of disease from one part to another; (3) mild
and not recurring; (4) excessive growth.

29. C11 **Biopsy** — (1) remove surgically; (2) sensation of dizziness; (3) removal of tissue for microscopic examination; (4) sign of disease.

30. C12 **Bladder** — (1) sac-like structure to collect protein; (2) another term for anus; (3) sac-like structure
storing bile; (4) sac-like structure collecting urine.

31. A8 **Bradycardia** — (1) fast heartbeat; (2) slow heartbeat; (3) irregular heartbeat; (4) heart defective
A10   from birth.

32. C13 **Bronchi** — (1) right and left windpipes entering lungs; (2) tube carrying oxygen to heart; (3) tube
taking food to stomach; (4) abnormal growth.

33. C13 **Bronchial Endoscope** — instrument used to (1) open bronchi; (2) photograph bronchi; (3) remove
D1   congestion; (4) look inside bronchi.
C28

34. C13 **Bronchoscopy** — (1) puncture of bronchi; (2) examination of bronchi with special instrument; (3)
D22   picture of bronchi; (4) removal of bronchi.

35. C14 **Calculus** — (1) vary from normal; (2) the brain; (3) a stone; (4) the small intestine.

36. C15 **Cancer** — (1) existing at birth; (2) organ in stomach; (3) malignant tumor; (4) shifting of disease
          from one part to another.

37. A9   **Carcinoma** — (1) malignant tumor; (2) extraction of cancer; (3) shifting of disease from one part to
     D17   another; (4) enlarged growth of the pancreas.

38. C16 **Cardiac Arrest** — (1) stoppage of heart; (2) heart attack; (3) stroke; (4) electric charge given heart
          to restart beating.

39. A10 **Cardiology** — is the science of the (1) lungs; (2) bronchi; (3) heart; (4) nervous system.
     D16

40. A11 **Cauterization** — (1) destroy tissue by burning; (2) vessel contraction; (3) symptoms occurring
     D24   together; (4) separation of vessels.

41. C17 **Cephalgia** — (1) backache; (2) earache; (3) sore throat; (4) headache.
     D2

42. C17 **Cephalic** — (1) picture of head; (2) cutting operation on head; (3) relating to head; (4) relating to ap-
     D8   pendix.

43. C17 **Cephalus** — (1) the front of the head; (2) the entire head; (3) the lungs; (4) the back of the head.

44. C18 **Cerebral** — (1) relating to the brain; (2) the skull; (3) the brain covering; (4) the spinal cord.
     D1

45. C18 **Cerebral Hemorrhage** — (1) bursting of brain blood vessel; (2) jarring injury to the brain; (3) loss of
     D1   oxygen to the liver; (4) picture of the brain.
     A39, D19

46. C18 **Cerebrum** — (1) side of brain controlling breathing; (2) entire brain; (3) front of the brain; (4) major
          brain vessel.

47. A12 **Cholecystectomy** — (1) removal of cyst from colon; (2) removal of appendix; (3) removal of gall
     C23   bladder; (4) removal of pancreas.
     D4

48. A12 **Cholelithiasis** — (1) formation of gall stones; (2) removal of gall stones; (3) instrument for viewing
     C40   gall bladder; (4) fluid produced by gall bladder.
     D25

49. A13 **Chondritis** — (1) painful nerves; (2) inflammation of cartilage; (3) headache; (4) vessel cramp.
     D10

50. A14 **Chronic** — (1) relating to chest; (2) relating to stomach; (3) short duration; (4) recurring frequently.
     D8

51. C19 **Clean** — (1) to remove surgically; (2) free of pus-producing germs; (3) limited area of the body; (4)
          free of all living germs.

52. C20 **Colon** — (1) liver; (2) kidney; (3) small intestine; (4) large intestine.

53. C20 **Colostomy** — (1) operation to make permanent hole in large intestine; (2) removal of small in-
    D27   testine; (3) cutting off kidney; (4) removal of tumor in pancreas.

54. C21 **Coma** — (1) deep unconsciousness; (2) state of hypnotic sleep; (3) brain stroke; (4) loss of oxygen in brain.

55. A15 **Concussion** — (1) blood clot; (2) injury to lungs; (3) injury to the brain; (4) large intestine.
    D24

56. A16 **Congenital** — (1) acquired after birth; (2) defective genes; (3) defect in genital area of body; (4) ex-
    D1   isting at birth.

57. A17 **Contusion** — (1) laceration; (2) bruise; (3) injury to brain; (4) large intestine.
    D24

58. A18 **Convulsion** — (1) nausea; (2) irregular body movements; (3) loss of air; (4) dizziness.
    D24

59. A19 **Coronary Thrombosis** — (1) stroke; (2) irregular heartbeat; (3) heart attack due to clot in the coro-
    C63   nary vessels; (4) heart attack due to clot in the aorta.
    D25

60. C22 **Cranial** — (1) skull fracture; (2) arm bone; (3) relating to the skull; (4) picture of the skull.
    D1

61. C22 **Cranium** — (1) the brain; (2) the skull; (3) the cerebrum; (4) the medulla.

62. C22 **Craniotomy** — (1) brain surgery; (2) cutting the skull; (3) prefrontal lobotomy; (4) brain concus-
    D27   sion.

63. A20 **Cyanosis** — (1) removal of cyst from lung; (2) formation of cyanic acid in stomach; (3) blue ap-
    D25   pearance of skin due to anoxia; (4) loss of appetite.

64. C23 **Cyst** — (1) bladder-like sac containing fluid; (2) area of diseased tissue; (3) crack in bone; (4) sud-den drop in blood pressure.

65. C23 **Cystocele** — (1) cells from tumor on bladder; (2) cells from stomach tumors; (3) protrusion of
    D14   stomach; (4) protrusion of bladder.

66. C23 **Cystoscopy** — (1) instrument examination of bladder; (2) picture of tumor in bladder; (3) scrap-
    D22   pings of cells from bladder; (4) removal of bladder.

67. A21 **Defibrillation** — (1) slow respiration; (2) remove gall stone; (3) empty stomach; (4) slow heartbeat
    C31, D24   electrically.

68. A22 **Dermatoid** — (1) skin tear; (2) resembling skin; (3) stitch to hold wound closed; (4) sac containing
    D15   fluid.

69. A22 **Dermatoma** — (1) glandular tissue; (2) headache; (3) skin tumor; (4) skin tear.
    D17

70. A23 **Diagnosis** — (1) loss of appetite; (2) identification of a condition; (3) forecast of recovery; (4) front
    D5   surface of the body.

71. C24 **Dirty** — (1) stained slide; (2) stone; (3) fused membrane; (4) containing pus-producing germs.

72. C25 **Disease** — (1) tear in skin; (2) sickness; (3) injury; (4) stitch to hold wound closed.

73. A24 **Distal** — (1) part of limb furthest from trunk; (2) back surface of body; (3) front surface of body; (4)
    D1   entire surface of body.

74. A25 **Dorsal** — (1) front surface of body; (2) part of limb nearest trunk; (3) back surface of body; (4) en-
    D1   tire surface of body.

75. A27 **Dysmenorrhea** — (1) hemorrhage from bladder; (2) hemorrhage from intestine; (3) painful flow of
    D19   monthly menses; (4) lack of monthly menses.

76. A26 **Dyspnea** — (1) spitting up blood; (2) difficulty breathing due to blocked airway; (3) shallow
    D21   breathing; (4) irregular breathing.

77. A26 **Dysuria** — (1) long menses flow; (2) painful urination; (3) stoppage of menses; (4) blood in urine.
    D25

78. C26 **Eclampsia** — (1) caesarean section; (2) regular childbirth; (3) loss of baby due to hemorrhage during
                  birth; (4) convulsion before or after delivery.

79. A28 **Ectopic** — (1) occurring outside the body; (2) inside body surface; (3) having poor eyesight; (4) oc-
    D8   curring in likely place.

80. C27 **Edema** — (1) fluid in abdominal cavity; (2) overbreathing; (3) irregular heartbeat; (4) fluid in the
                  tissue.

81. A29 **Embolism** — (1) vary from normal; (2) tumor on a stem; (3) tear in skin; (4) blocking of vessel by a
    D9   traveling blood clot.

82. A30 **Encephalography** — is a picture of (1) outside of skull; (2) spinal column; (3) inside of head; (4)
    C17   brain vessel transplant.
    D6

83. A31 **Endotracheal** — (1) to cut into trachea; (2) to take a picture of trachea; (3) relating to inside of
    C65   trachea; (4) relating to area around trachea.
    D1

84. A32 **Enteritis** — (1) inflammation of stomach; (2) inflammation of intestine; (3) hole in large intestine;
    D10   (4) tumor on large intestine.

85. A32 **Enterostomy** — (1) cutting away of intestine; (2) puncture intestine to let out fluid; (3) make perma-
    D27   nent opening in intestine; (4) close punctured intestine.

86. A33 **Entopic** — (1) abnormal; (2) occurring in normal place; (3) outside of body; (4) side of body.
    D8

87. C29 **Epistaxis** — (1) loss of vision; (2) loss of hearing; (3) nosebleed; (4) paralysis of upper part of body.

88. C30 **Esophageal Endoscope** — (1) instrument used to look inside esophagus; (2) instrument used to cut
D1   open esophagus; (3) machine to photograph esophagus; (4) puncture
C28   esophagus to release air.

89. C30 **Esophagoscopy** — (1) removal of esophagus; (2) picture of esophagus; (3) transplant of esophagus;
D22   (4) examination of esophagus with instrument.

90. C30 **Esophagus** — (1) tube from mouth to lung; (2) tube from mouth to stomach; (3) tube from kidney
            to stomach; (4) tube from mouth to nose.

91. A34 **Excision** — (1) rapid examination of tissue; (2) fast heartbeat; (3) tube from kidney to bladder; (4)
D24   remove by cutting out.

92. C31 **Fibrillation** — (1) fast respiration; (2) fast heartbeat; (3) gall stones in liver; (4) over-eat.
D24

93. A35 **Fibroid** — (1) resembling fibrous tissue; (2) tear in fibroid; (3) large intestine; (4) area of diseased
D15   tissue.

94. A35 **Fibroma** — (1) vessel cramp; (2) tumor of the nerves; (3) contraction of the stomach; (4) fibrous
D17   tumor.

95. C32 **Fracture** — (1) drooping of an organ; (2) crack in a bone; (3) a tissue growth with no purpose; (4)
           stone.

96. A36 **Frozen Section** — (1) rapid examination of tissue; (2) heart stoppage; (3) surgical tissue removal for
D23   examination; (4) dislodged blood clot.

97. A37 **Gall Bladder** — (1) sac that stores insulin; (2) sac that stores bile; (3) sac that stores sugar; (4) organ
C12   that produces starch.

98. A38 **Gastralgia** — (1) gas in intestine; (2) painful chest; (3) painful kidney; (4) painful stomach.
D2

99. A38 **Gastroenteritis** — (1) inflammation of stomach and intestine; (2) removal of stomach ulcers; (3) in-
A32   flammation of intestine; (4) hole in stomach wall.
D10

100. C33 **Heart** — (1) organ used in thinking; (2) generosity; (3) muscular organ between lungs; (4) organ in
           stomach.

101. A39 **Hematology** — (1) blood transfusion; (2) shortage of oxygen in the blood; (3) science of the blood;
D16   (4) bursting of a blood vessel.

102. A40 **Hemoptysis** — (1) bleeding from lungs; (2) brain hemorrhage; (3) vessel cramp; (4) multiple
D25   hemorrhaging.

103. A39 **Hemorrhage** — (1) bursting of the gall bladder; (2) bursting forth of blood; (3) inflammation of the
D19   aorta; (4) procedure to obtain blood count.

104. A41 **Hepatitis** — (1) inflammation of the liver; (2) inflammation of the kidney; (3) broken intestine lin-
D10   ing; (4) intestinal strangulation.

105. C34 **Hernia** — (1) protrusion of an organ through wall or cavity; (2) falling of an organ; (3) painful
nerves; (4) limited body area.

106. A42 **Hydrocele** — (1) water in bladder; (2) electric shock treatment; (3) excess water in stomach; (4)
D14   water hernia in testicle.

107. A42 **Hydroencephalograph** — (1) to take water from the brain; (2) fluid pressure of brain; (3) picture of
A30   water inside head; (4) fluid draining from skull.
C17, D6

108. A43 **Hypertrophy** — (1) degeneration of body part; (2) excessive growth of body part; (3) severe and
D28   recurring; (4) mild and not recurring.

109. A43 **Hyperventilation** — (1) sensation of dizziness; (2) fainting; (3) overbreathing; (4) difficulty of
B29   breathing due to blocked air passage.
D24

110. A44 **Hysteropexy** — (1) removal of uterus; (2) another term for hysterectomy; (3) fastening of uterus in
D20   place; (4) caesarian section.

111. A44 **Hysterotomy** — (1) operation to control hysteria; (2) cutting of uterus; (3) removal of uterus; (4) in-
D27   strument examination of uterus.

112. C35 **Ileostomy** — (1) cutting to make permanent opening in small intestine; (2) removal of ileum; (3)
D27   picture of ileum; (4) instrument used to look into brain.

113. C35 **Ileum** — (1) kidney; (2) bladder; (3) small intestine; (4) large intestine.

114. B1   **Internal** — (1) the part of the body away from surface; (2) the digestive tract; (3) the respiratory
D1   system; (4) surface of the body.

115. C36 **Intestine** — (1) stomach; (2) lower digestive tract; (3) liver; (4) anus.

116. C37 **Kidney** — (1) organ manufacturing urine; (2) organ producing bile; (3) organ digesting starches; (4)
organ used for feeding baby.

117. B2   **Laceration** — (1) drop in blood pressure; (2) removal of lung; (3) tear in skin; (4) relating to the
D24   head.

118. B2   **Laparotomy** — (1) to remove liver; (2) insert tube into stomach; (3) picture of abdomen; (4) to cut
D27   into the abdomen.

119. B4   **Laryngospasm** — (1) muscle contraction of voice box; (2) removal of voice box; (3) tumor on
D26   larynx; (4) puncture in muscle of voice box.

120. C38 **Lesion** — (1) growth of tissue with no purpose; (2) stitch to close a wound; (3) area of diseased
tissue; (4) cracked bone.

121. C39 **Liver** — (1) organ producing protein; (2) organ removing waste; (3) organ producing bile; (4) organ
producing plasma.

122. B5 **Local** — (1) specific area of body; (2) single organ in chest; (3) particular muscle in arm; (4) opera-
    D1   tion on abdomen.

123. C41 **Lungs** — (1) balloon-like structures in chest; (2) organ which digests food; (3) organ which pumps
blood; (4) organ removing solid waste.

124. C42 **Malaise** — (1) bursting of blood vessel in the brain; (2) vague feeling of illness; (3) sign of disease;
(4) injury.

125. C43 **Malignant** — (1) severe, growing worse; (2) not fatal; (3) mild and not recurring; (4) synonym for
ulcerous growth.

126. C44 **Meninges** — (1) fluid brain floats in; (2) gray matter in brain; (3) convolutions in cerebrum; (4)
brain covering.

127. C44 **Meningitis** — (1) inflammation of skull; (2) inflammation of spinal cord; (3) inflammation of brain
    D10   blood vessels; (4) inflammation of brain covering.

128. C44 **Meningocele** — (1) herniation of brain covering; (2) herniation of skull covering; (3) cell in brain;
    D14   (4) slides of brain cells.

129. B6 **Menopause** — (1) decrease in flow of menses; (2) stoppage of monthly menses flow; (3) increase in
    D18   menses; (4) infantile pregnancy.

130. B6 **Menorrhagia** — (1) stoppage of menses flow; (2) hemorrhage of the uterus; (3) infrequent menses
    D19   flow; (4) excessive menstrual flow.

131. B7 **Metastasis** — (1) many parts of body; (2) changes undergone by fertilized human egg; (3) the shift-
    D25   ing of disease from one part of the body to another; (4) malignant tumor.

132. B7 **Metastatic** — (1) many body parts; (2) stage in egg fertilization process; (3) relating to disease shift-
    D8   ing through body; (4) malignant tumor.

133. B9 **Myelography** — (1) picture of the head; (2) picture of the stomach; (3) picture of the spinal cord; (4)
    D6   picture of the liver.

134. B8 **Myoid** — (1) muscle-like; (2) inflammation of a joint; (3) vessel cramp; (4) kidney transplant.
    D15

135. B8 **Myoma** — (1) bursting blood vessel; (2) painful nerve; (3) growth of useless tissue; (4) muscle
    D17   tumor.

136. C45 **Neoplasm** — (1) injury; (2) growth of tissue with no purpose; (3) drooping of organ; (4) stone.

137. B10 **Nephropexy** — (1) operation to fasten kidney in place; (2) removal of kidney; (3) kidney transplant;
    D20   (4) examination of kidney.

138. B10 **Nephrostomy** — (1) operation to make permanent opening in kidney; (2) removal of kidney; (3)
     D27 kidney transplant; (4) examination of kidney.

139. B11 **Neuralgia** — (1) painful joints; (2) headache; (3) fainting; (4) painful nerves.
     D2

140. B11 **Neurology** — (1) science of the heart; (2) tissue scraping; (3) fainting; (4) science of the nerves.
     D16

141. B12 **Oophorectomy** — (1) removal of kidney; (2) removal of ovary; (3) removal of ureter; (4) removal
     D4 of testicle.

142. B13 **Orchidotomy** — (1) removal of tube from ovary to uterus; (2) removal of kidney; (3) surgery on
     D27 testicle; (4) removal of large intestine.

143. B13 **Orchitis** — (1) inflammation of large intestine; (2) removal of large intestine; (3) inflammation of
     D10 testicle; (4) inflammation of vagina.

144. B14 **Osteitis** — (1) inflammation of eye; (2) inflammation of bone; (3) blood clot; (4) area of diseased
     D10 tissue.

145. C46 **Ovary** — (1) human egg; (2) male sex gland; (3) gland producing bile; (4) sex gland producing egg.

146. B15 **Paracentesis** — (1) puncture of organs alongside cavity to release fluid; (2) form of paralysis; (3)
     D3 stroke; (4) bursting of a blood vessel.

147. C47 **Pelvic** — (1) relating to sexual intercourse; (2) backside of body; (3) relating to pelvis; (4) to cut
     D8 pelvis to release fluid.

148. C47 **Pelvis** — (1) female sex organ; (2) basin-shaped bones of lower trunk; (3) male sex organ; (4)
female sex hormone.

149. B16 **Perianal** — (1) around large intestine; (2) diseased anus; (3) enlarged anus; (4) tissue around anus.
     C6

150. B17 **Peripheral** — (1) outside head; (2) outside hair on body; (3) infected area outside body surface; (4)
     D1 related to the outside of the body.

151. B18 **Peritonitis** — (1) inflammation of lining inside abdomen; (2) inflammation of anus lining; (3) in-
     D10 flammation of large intestine; (4) infection of small intestine.

152. B19 **Pneumonectomy** — (1) removal of bronchi; (2) removal of lung; (3) removal of heart; (4) removal
     D4 of windpipe.

153. B19 **Pneumonia** — (1) picture of lung; (2) relating to the lung; (3) inflammation of chest; (4) inflamma-
     D7 tion of the lung.

154. B19 **Pneumonitis** — (1) inflammation of the chest; (2) congestion in lung; (3) pneumonia; (4) too little
     D10 oxygen in lung.

155. B19 **Pneumothorax** — (1) hole in lung; (2) blood in lung; (3) bursting of blood vessel in lung; (4) sudden
     C62 collapse of lung.

156. C48 **Polyp** — (1) tumor on a stem; (2) stitch to close a wound; (3) painful stomach; (4) instrumental exam of kidney.

157. B21 **Proctoscopy** — (1) instrumental exam of intestine; (2) instrumental exam of rectum; (3) instrumental exam of liver; (4) instrumental exam of kidney.
    D22

158. B20 **Prognosis** — (1) blue appearance of skin; (2) the entire body; (3) muscle tumor; (4) forecast of condition.
    D5

159. C49 **Prostate** — (1) tube carrying urine in body; (2) operation for removal of ovary; (3) tube from kidney to bladder; (4) gland surrounding bladder.

160. C49 **Prostatectomy** — (1) removal of prostate; (2) enlargement of prostate; (3) puncture of prostate; (4) picture of prostate.
    D4

161. B22 **Proximal** — (1) part of limb furthest from trunk; (2) part of limb nearest trunk; (3) back body surface; (4) front body surface.
    D1

162. B23 **Ptosis** — (1) sudden drop in blood pressure; (2) painful nerves; (3) fainting; (4) drooping of an organ.
    D25

163. C50 **Radical Resection** — (1) examination of diseased tissue; (2) tear in skin; (3) injury to the brain; (4) surgical removal of organ and surrounding parts.

164. C51 **Rectocele** — (1) protrustion of rectum; (2) cells located in rectum; (3) hole in rectum; (4) puncture of rectum to let out air.
    D14

165. C51 **Rectum** — (1) large intestine; (2) last part of large intestine; (3) end of small intestine; (4) extra bone in chest.

166. C52 **Septic** — (1) free of pus-producing germs; (2) free of all living germs; (3) containing pus-producing germs; (4) containing living germs.

167. C53 **Shock** — (1) drop in heartbeat; (2) shallow breathing; (3) too little oxygen in blood; (4) drop in blood pressure.

168. C54 **Sterile** — (1) free of pus-producing germs; (2) free of all living germs; (3) fluid that kills germs; (4) limited infected area.

169. C55 **Stomach** — (1) organ that digests food; (2) organ that removes sugar from food; (3) stretchy organ for collection of swallowed food; (4) organ that breaks down food into protein.

170. C56 **Stroke** — (1) heart attack; (2) brain concussion; (3) blood in lungs; (4) bursting of blood vessel in brain.

171. C57 **Suture** — (1) abnormal sticking together; (2) stitch to hold wound closed; (3) area of diseased tissue; (4) crack in bone.

172. C58 **Symptom** — (1) loss of appetite; (2) fluid in tissue; (3) area of diseased tissue; (4) sign of disease.

173. C59 **Syncope** — (1) dizziness; (2) fainting; (3) loss of appetite; (4) over-breathing.

174. C60 **Syndrome** — (1) painful nerves; (2) drop in blood pressure; (3) group of symptoms occurring together; (4) forecast of recovery.

175. B24 **Systemic** — (1) relating to the entire body; (2) blood system; (3) nervous system; (4) digestive
D8   system.

176. B25 **Tachycardia** — (1) irregular heartbeat; (2) heart with birth defect; (3) too little oxygen in heart; (4)
A10   fast heartbeat.

177. B26 **Tenontitis** — (1) inflammation of the tendon; (2) inflammation of the bone; (3) inflammation of the
D10   cartilage; (4) blocked windpipe.

178. C61 **Testicle** — (1) female sex gland; (2) passage tube to penis from kidney; (3) producer of human
zygote; (4) male sex gland.

179. C62 **Thoracentesis** — (1) picture of windpipe; (2) puncture thorax to release air; (3) puncture stomach to
D3   let out fluid; (4) removal of lung.

180. C62 **Thoracic** — (1) relating to the thorax; (2) to take a picture of the thorax; (3) relating to the lungs; (4)
D8   inflammation of the thorax.

181. C62 **Thoracotomy** — (1) to remove thorax; (2) cut thorax; (3) puncture thorax to let out air; (4) take
D27   picture of thorax.

182. C62 **Thorax** — (1) windpipe; (2) bronchial tubes; (3) lungs; (4) bony cage of chest.

183. C63 **Thrombus** — (1) bloodclot; (2) stroke; (3) heart attack; (4) bursting of vessel due to high blood
pressure.

184. C64 **Thyroid** — (1) gland near upper part of trachea; (2) gland near sinus cavity; (3) gland near small intestine; (4) gland in eyes.

185. C64 **Thyroidectomy** — (1) picture of thyroid; (2) removal of thyroid; (3) irregular growth of thyroid; (4)
D4   puncture of thyroid to release fluid.

186. C65 **Trachea** — (1) tube from nose to mouth; (2) tube from mouth to lungs; (3) tube from throat to
mouth; (4) tube from lungs to heart.

187. C65 **Tracheal Endoscope** — (1) pictures of tracheal wall; (2) laboratory scraping of inside trachea; (3) in-
D1   strument to look inside trachea; (4) puncture trachea.
C28

188. C65 **Tracheoscopy** — (1) examination of trachea with special instrument; (2) puncture trachea; (3)
D22   operation on trachea for examination; (4) puncture trachea by accident.

189. C65 **Tracheotomy** — (1) remove trachea; (2) transplant artificial trachea; (3) close up hole in trachea; (4)
D27   cutting operation on trachea.

190. C66 **Trauma** — (1) injury; (2) protrusion of the rectum; (3) organ manufacture; (4) sudden drop in
blood pressure.

191. C67 **Tumor** — (1) growth of tissue with no purpose; (2) area of diseased tissue; (3) stone; (4) large intestine.

192. B27 **Unsterile** — (1) not free of all living germs; (2) not free of all pus-producing germs; (3) containing
    C67 fluid or air; (4) water that contains metal.

193. C68 **Ureter** — (1) tube from liver to bladder; (2) tube from kidney to bladder; (3) tube from small intestine to liver; (4) another word for liver.

194. C68 **Ureterotomy** — (1) removal of ureter; (2) puncture of ureter to release fluid; (3) cutting operation
    D27 on ureter; (4) enlargement of ureter.

195. C69 **Urethra** — (1) tube carrying egg to womb; (2) tube carrying urine outside body; (3) anesthetic to aid sleep; (4) female hormone.

196. C69 **Urethritis** — (1) removal of urethra; (2) extraction of urethra by x-ray; (3) enlargement of urethra;
    D10 (4) inflammation of urethra.

197. C70 **Uterus** — (1) pear-shaped organ called womb; (2) passage way to womb; (3) cavity womb rests in; (4) tube from kidney to womb.

198. C71 **Vagina** — (1) female organ of sexual intercourse; (2) afterbirth; (3) another term for womb; (4) cutting operation on ureter.

199. C71 **Vaginitis** — (1) removal of vagina; (2) swelling of vagina; (3) inflammation of vagina; (4) cutting
    D10 operation on vagina.

200. B28 **Vasospasm** — (1) vessel cramp; (2) muscle cramp; (3) painful neck; (4) painful joints.
    D26

201. C72 **Ventral** — (1) front surface of the body; (2) back of the body; (3) top of the body; (4) right side of the body.

202. C73 **Vertigo** — (1) dizziness; (2) loss of appetite; (3) painful stomach; (4) free of all living germs.

Pre-test Answer Sheet

1. ___	27. ___	53. ___	79. ___	105. ___	131. ___	157. ___	180. ___
2. ___	28. ___	54. ___	80. ___	106. ___	132. ___	158. ___	181. ___
3. ___	29. ___	55. ___	81. ___	107. ___	133. ___	159. ___	182. ___
4. ___	30. ___	56. ___	82. ___	108. ___	134. ___	160. ___	183. ___
5. ___	31. ___	57. ___	83. ___	109. ___	135. ___	161. ___	184. ___
6. ___	32. ___	58. ___	84. ___	110. ___	136. ___	162. ___	185. ___
7. ___	33. ___	59. ___	85. ___	111. ___	137. ___	163. ___	186. ___
8. ___	34. ___	60. ___	86. ___	112. ___	138. ___	164. ___	187. ___
9. ___	35. ___	61. ___	87. ___	113. ___	139. ___	165. ___	188. ___
10. ___	36. ___	62. ___	88. ___	114. ___	140. ___	166. ___	189. ___
11. ___	37. ___	63. ___	89. ___	115. ___	141. ___	167. ___	190. ___
12. ___	38. ___	64. ___	90. ___	116. ___	142. ___	168. ___	191. ___
13. ___	39. ___	65. ___	91. ___	117. ___	143. ___	169. ___	192. ___
14. ___	40. ___	66. ___	92. ___	118. ___	144. ___	170. ___	193. ___
15. ___	41. ___	67. ___	93. ___	119. ___	145. ___	171. ___	194. ___
16. ___	42. ___	68. ___	94. ___	120. ___	146. ___	172. ___	195. ___
17. ___	43. ___	69. ___	95. ___	121. ___	147. ___	173. ___	196. ___
18. ___	44. ___	70. ___	96. ___	122. ___	148. ___	174. ___	197. ___
19. ___	45. ___	71. ___	97. ___	123. ___	149. ___	175. ___	198. ___
20. ___	46. ___	72. ___	98. ___	124. ___	150. ___	176. ___	199. ___
21. ___	47. ___	73. ___	99. ___	125. ___	151. ___	177. ___	200. ___
22. ___	48. ___	74. ___	100. ___	126. ___	152. ___	178. ___	201. ___
23. ___	49. ___	75. ___	101. ___	127. ___	153. ___	179. ___	202. ___
24. ___	50. ___	76. ___	102. ___	128. ___	154. ___		
25. ___	51. ___	77. ___	103. ___	129. ___	155. ___	SCORE ___________	
26. ___	52. ___	78. ___	104. ___	130. ___	156. ___		

Word/Picture Associations Keys to Memory

Now that you have completed the pre-test exercise you should have an accurate count of the number of words you need to learn. The various exercises that follow include all the words you have covered in the pre-test, the major differences being that the questions are presented in different formats and the words themselves are broken down into their several parts.

Most of these 202 words are made up of a prefix, a root (or whole word), and/or a suffix. As you study these words, you will find that certain prefixes and suffixes frequently reappear. For example, the suffix -al always means "relating to." By remembering this simple rule, you then can determine that intestinal (intestin[e]-al) means simply "relating to the intestines," and that tracheal (trache[a]-al) means "relating to the trachea."

Additionally, you will learn that a word which begins with the prefix derm- always has to do with the skin, and that a word beginning with the prefix cardi- always refers to the heart.

To assist you in learning all of these various prefixes, whole words, and suffixes, there follows a section of word/picture associations. These associations are broken down into the various parts of the words. Sections A and B contain all the prefixes used in the 202 words; Section C contains all the whole words; and Section D, all the suffixes. Attached to each word or word part there is a phonetic spelling of the word, followed by a brief definition. The picture, or cartoon, is designed to give you an easy-to-remember visual association for the word and its definition. The caption accompanying the cartoon contains the phonetic pronunciation of the word and its definition.

Look at association D1, page 98 of this book. The suffix is -al, which, as was noted before, means "related to." The cartoon with caption—"My Uncle Al is related to me."—is for your use as a memory association device. This particular association is clear-cut; others, due to the complexity of the word, are more difficult. If you find that some word/picture associations do not work for you, come up with another which you find easier to remember and more useful.

Before proceeding with the other exercises, turn back to the pre-test exercise. You will note that to the left of each word there is a number or list of numbers, each preceded by the letters A, B, C, or D. These letters and numbers refer you to the appropriate word/picture associations which will help you to learn and remember the meaning of each word.

For example, word number 3, abdominocentesis, refers you to associations C1 and D3. Turn to Section C (whole words) and look at association C1—abdomen. After studying the word, its definition, and the related cartoon and caption, turn to Section D (suffixes) and look at association D3—centesis—again studying the word, its definition, and cartoon and caption. You should now have a clear understanding of the meaning of the word, and hopefully the cartoon/memory device will enable you to retain the definition.

This procedure of looking up the word/picture associations for each of the words should be followed for all those words you did not know on the initial pre-test. As you go through the remaining exercises, you should repeat these steps for all those definitions you do not yet remember.

WORD/PICTURE ASSOCIATIONS

PREFIXES A

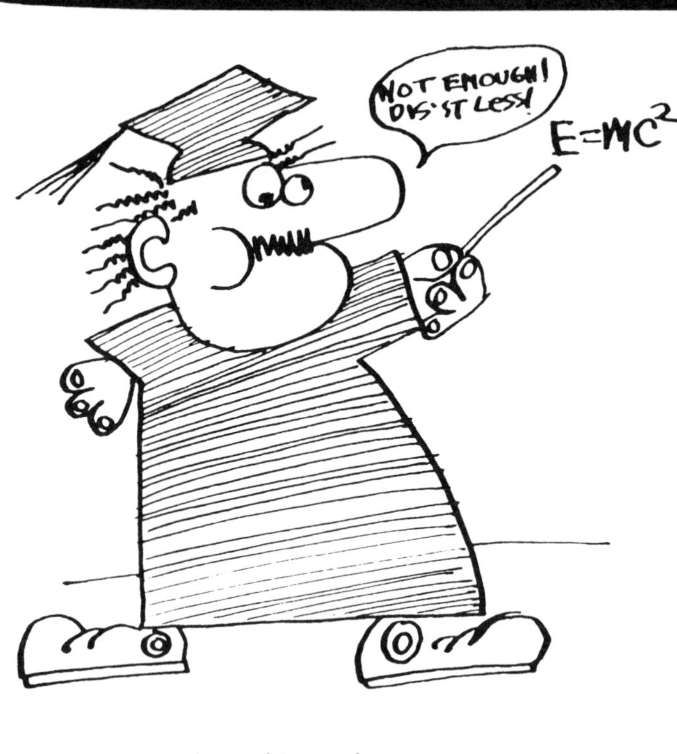

A-

not; without; lessen

A good **lesson** is **not**
without meaning.

A1

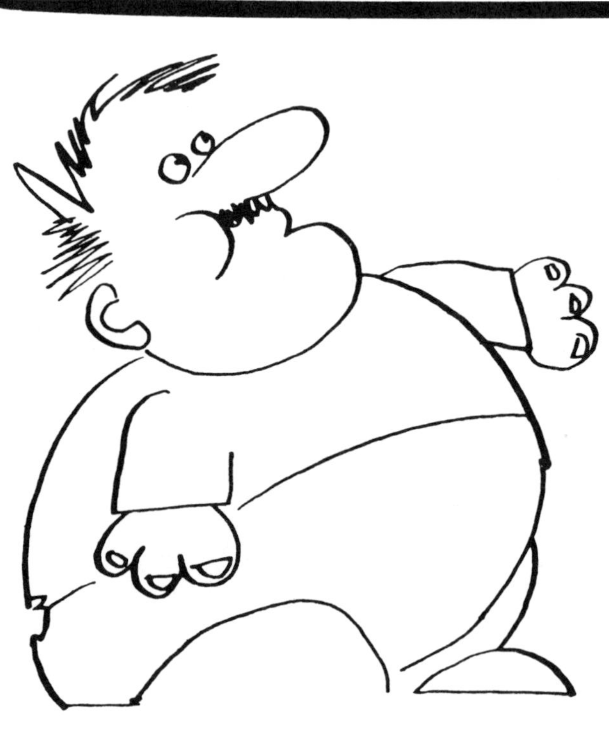

Aden-

add-en

gland; glandular
tissue

Add-no glandular tissue
to me; I'm fat enough.

A2

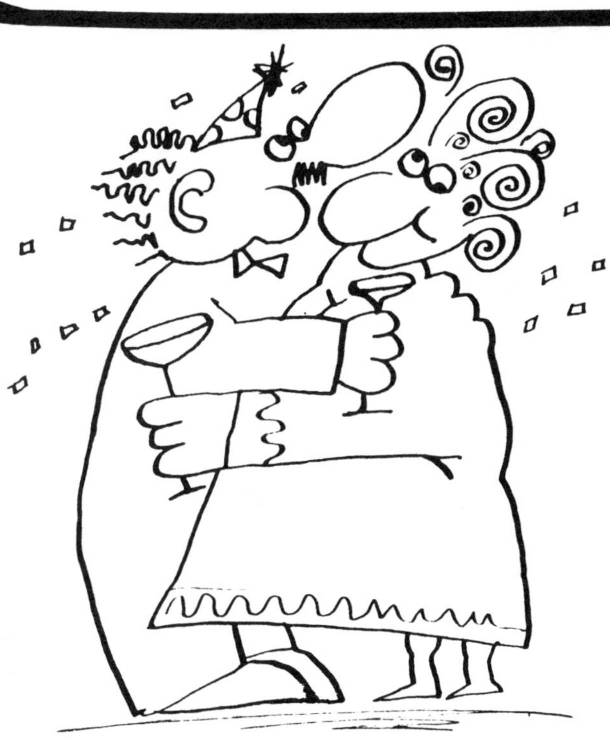

Adhe-

add-he

abnormal sticking
together

Had she and **Abe normally** planned to
be **sticking together** for New Year's Eve?

A3

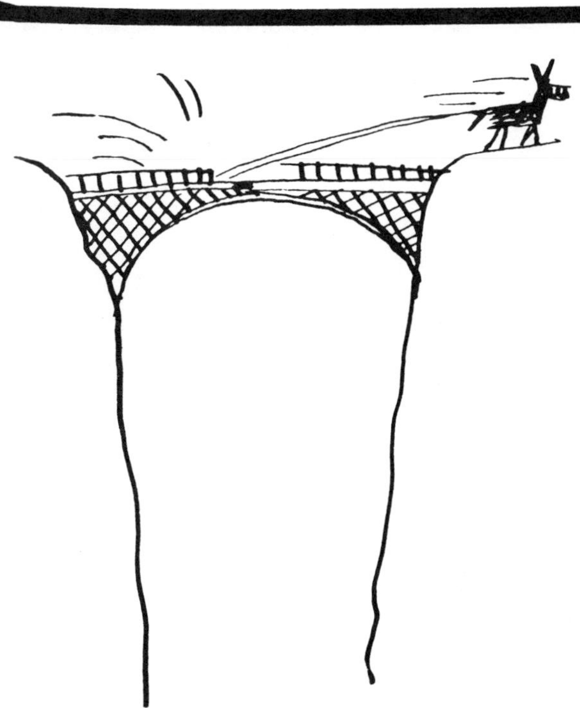

Anastomo-

ann-ass-tah-moh

join two parts to
make a new passageway

It took **an ass to move** the **two parts**
of the bridge into place.

A4

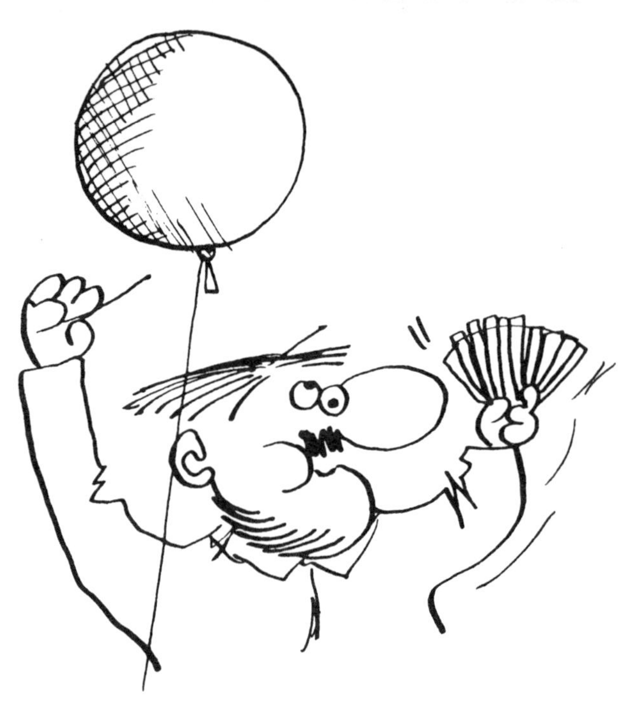

Aneury-

an-your

ballooning out of
blood vessel at
weak point

Fan your balloon outside; it makes my
blood sizzle and I'll bust it at a **weak point**.

A5

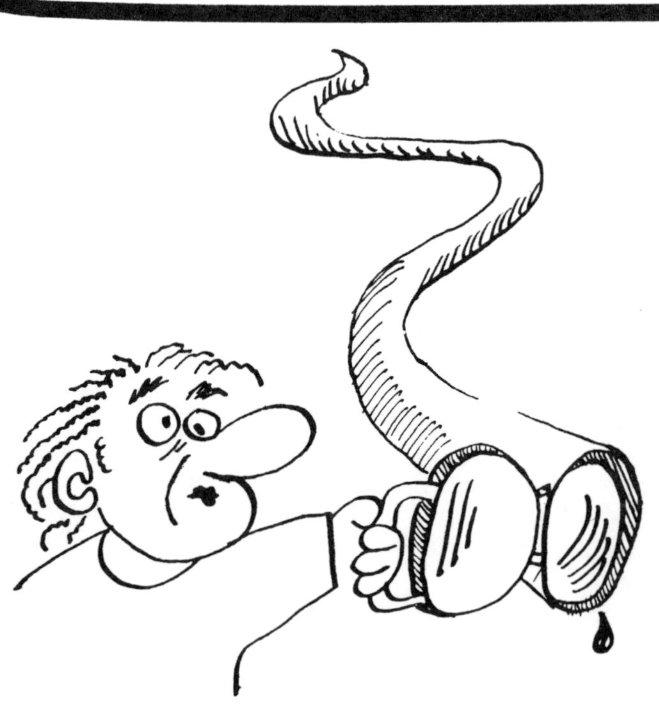

Angio-

ann-gee-o

blood vessel

Angie opened the **blood vessel,**
but nothing came out.

A6

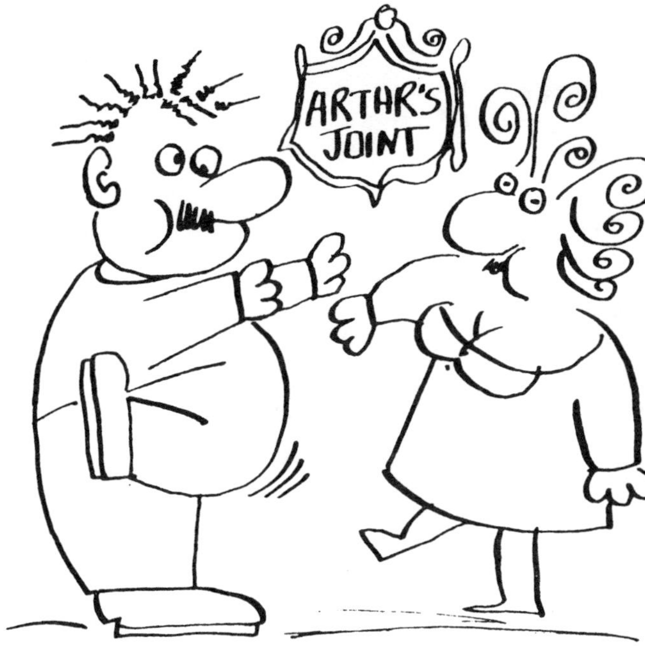

Arthur's is a **joint**
we go to dance in.

Arthr-

arth-r

joints

A7

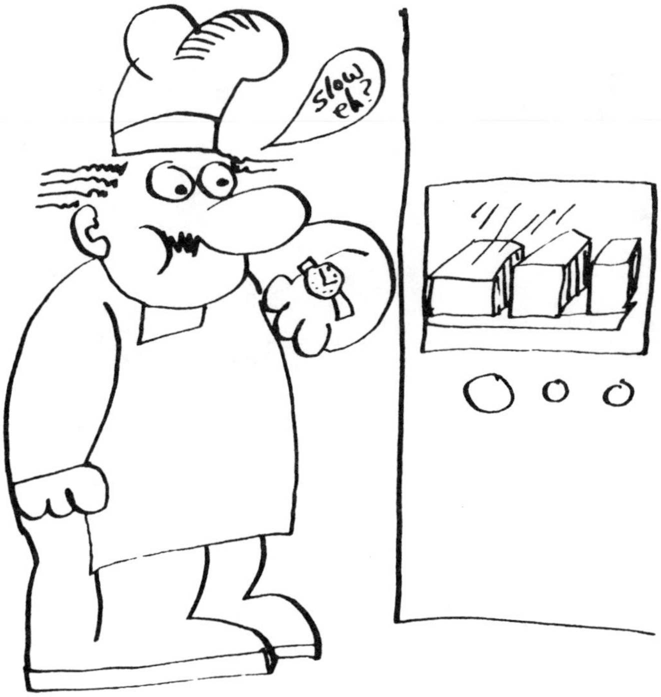

The **bread** bakes
very **slow**ly, **eh**?

Brady-

brad-eh

slow

A8

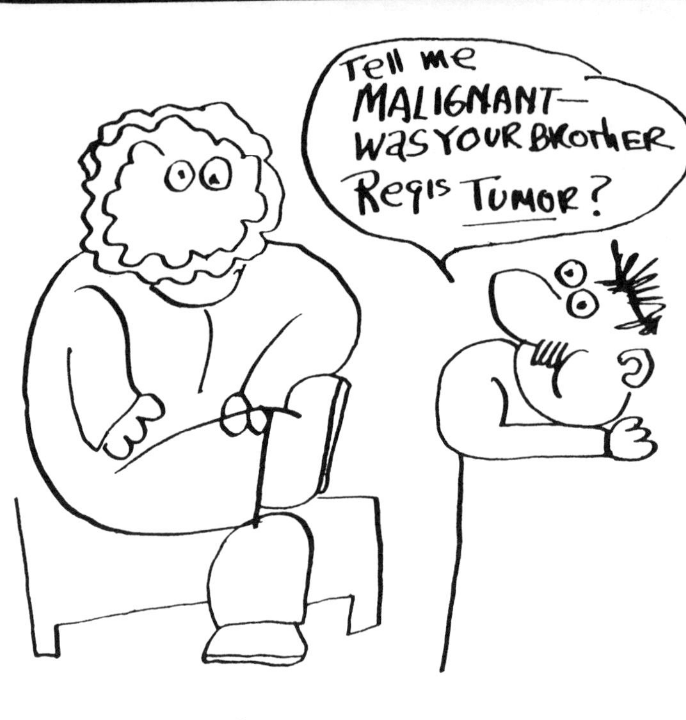

Carcin-

kar-sin

malignant

Johnny **Carson** never has a
malignant tumor on his show.

A9

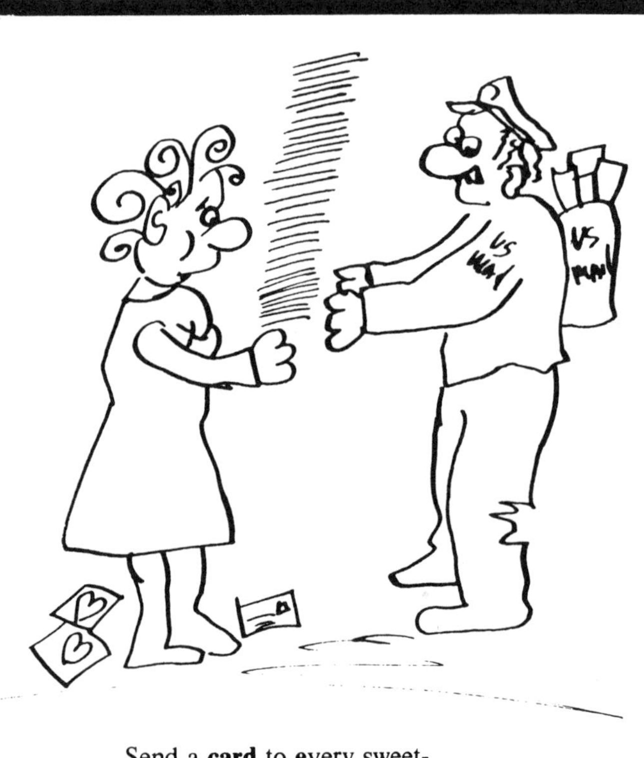

Cardi(a)-

car-dee-(a)

heart

Send a **card** to every sweet-
heart on Valentine's Day.

A10

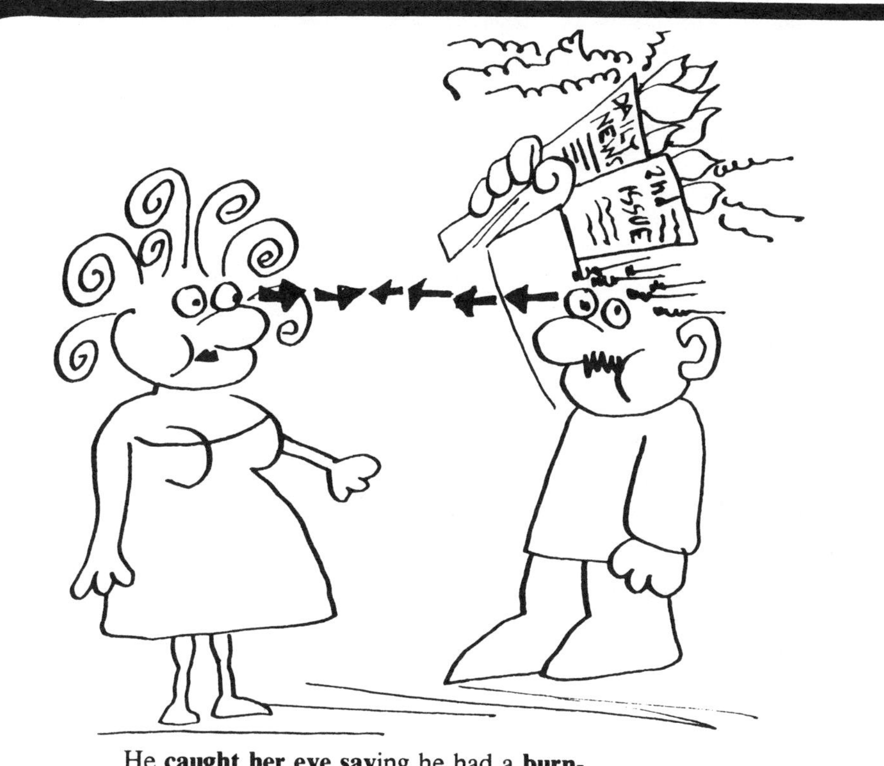

He **caught her eye** saying he had a **burn**-ing need to talk about curren**t issues**.

Cauteriza-

cau-ter-eye-zay

burn tissue

A11

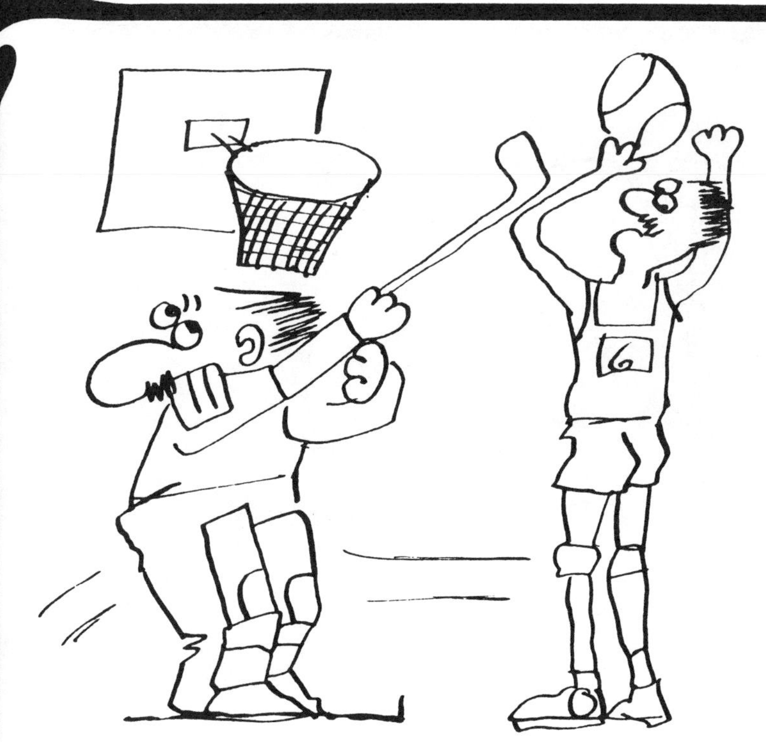

The **goalee** blocked the **ball** from going through the net.

Chole-

ko-lee

gall

A12

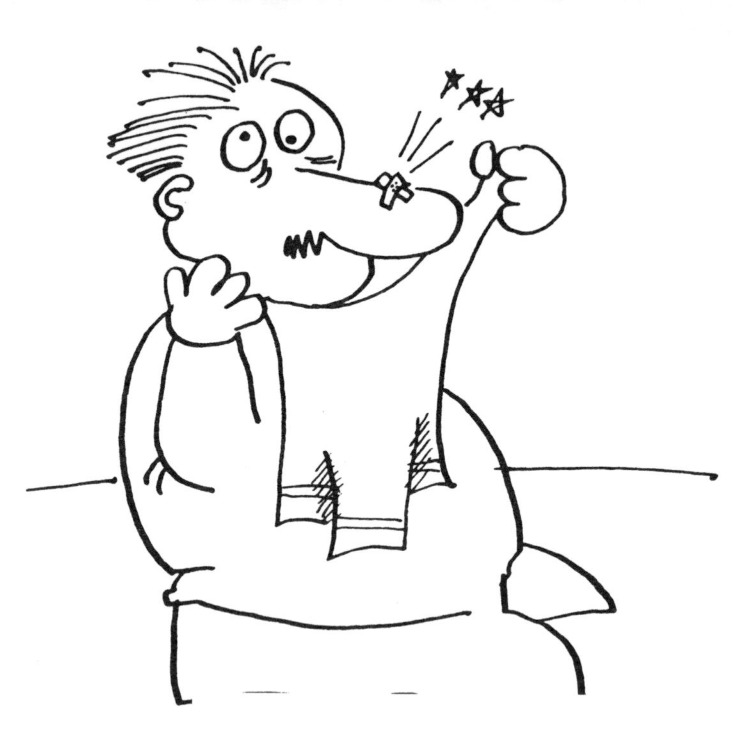

Chondri-

kon-dry

cartilage

You can dry your **cartilage** with a dish towel.

A13

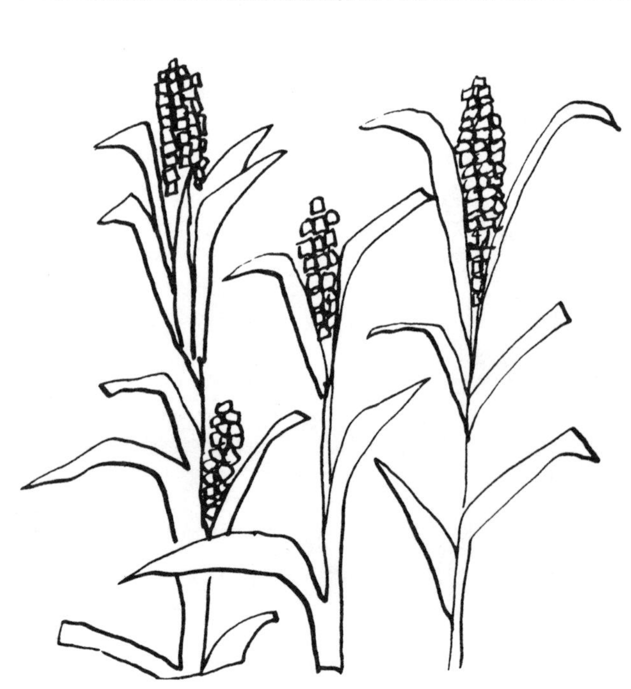

Chron-

kron

long duration; recurring frequently

Corn grows **slow**ly and has a long **maturation** period.

A14

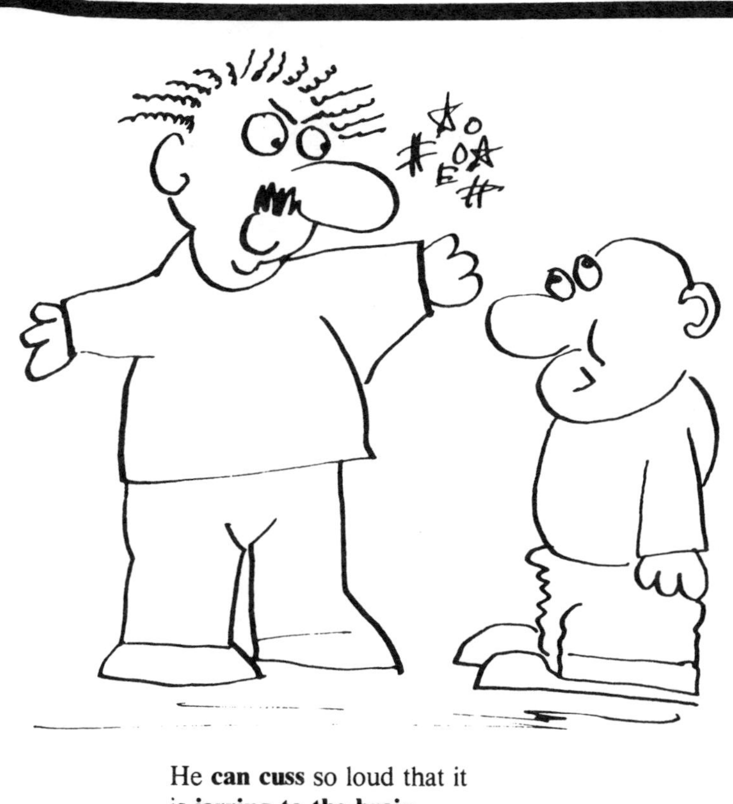

Concus-

kon-cuss

jarring injury
to the brain

He **can cuss** so loud that it
is **jarring to the brain**.

A15

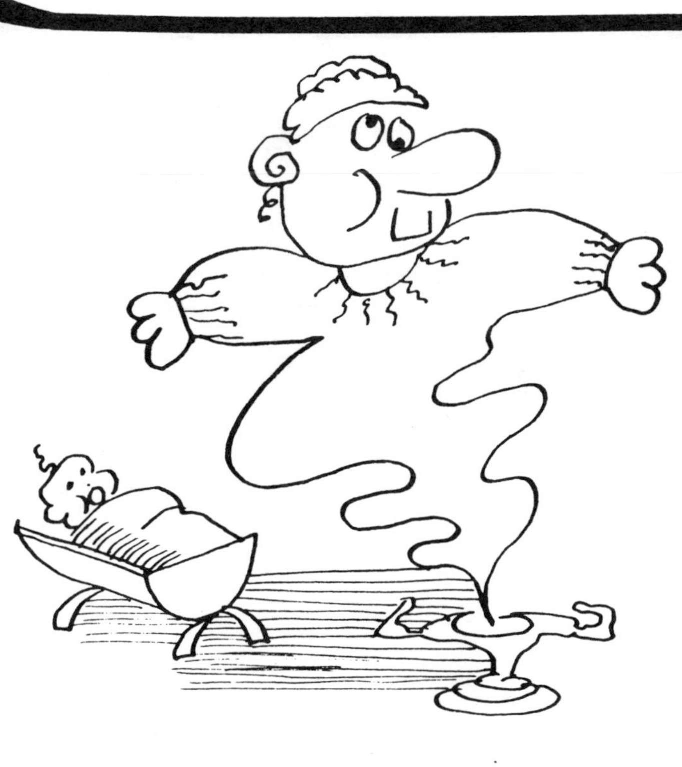

Congenit-

kon-gen-it

existing at birth

Can a geni tell you what **existed**
at the time you were **born**?

A16

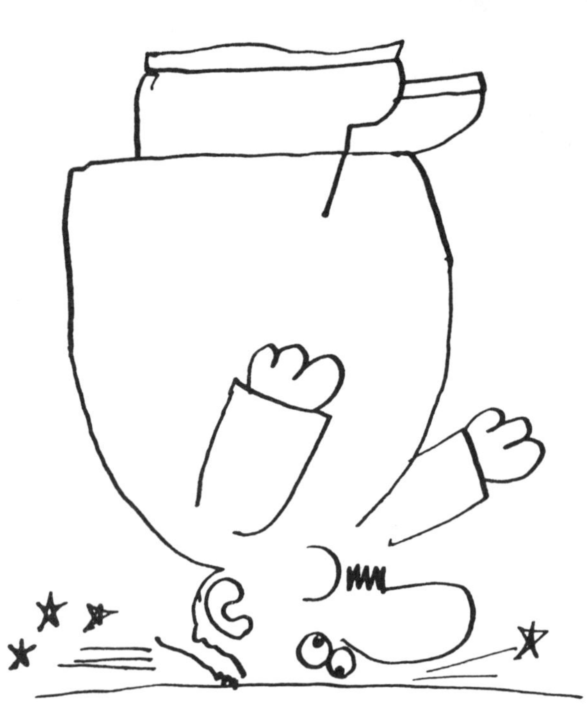

Contu-

kon-two

bruise

You can too bruise
your head by falling.

A17

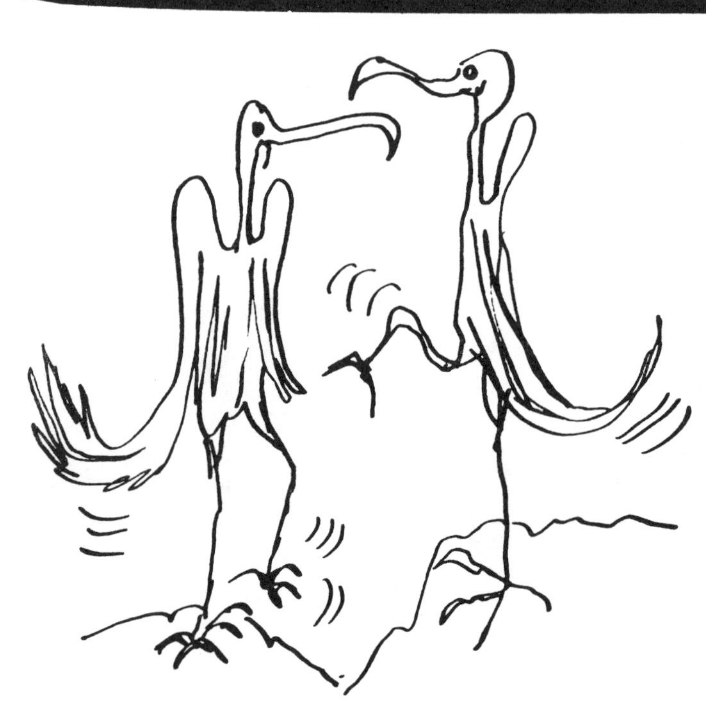

Convul-

kon-vull

irregular movements
of limbs

Condors and **vul**tures make **irregular
movements of limbs** and wings.

A18

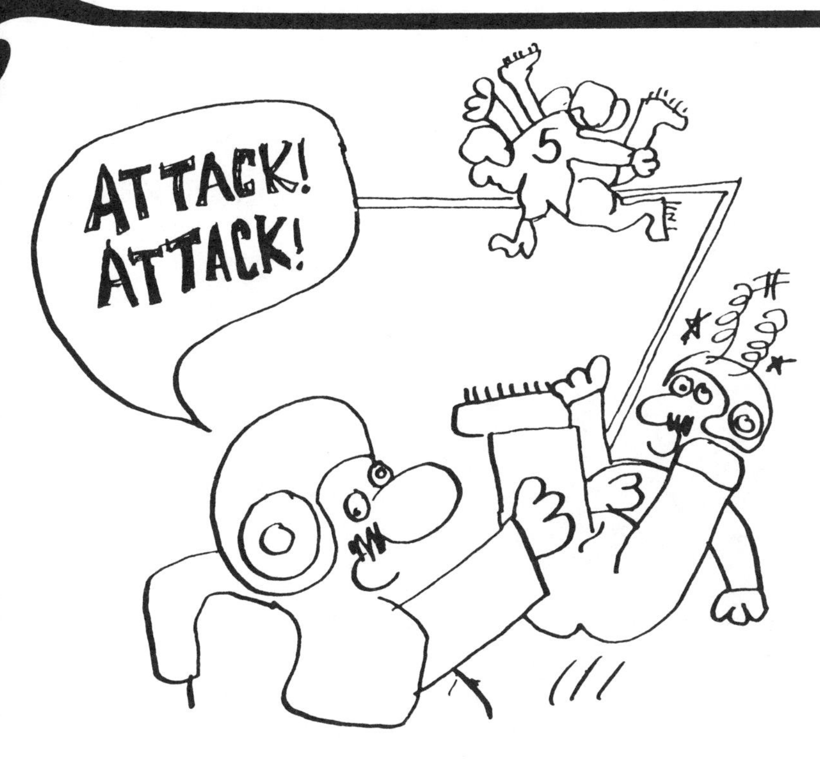

Coronary

kor-a-nar-ee

heart attack due
to blocked coronary
vessels

In football, I act **ornery** and **attack
heart**ily to **block corner hustles**.

A19

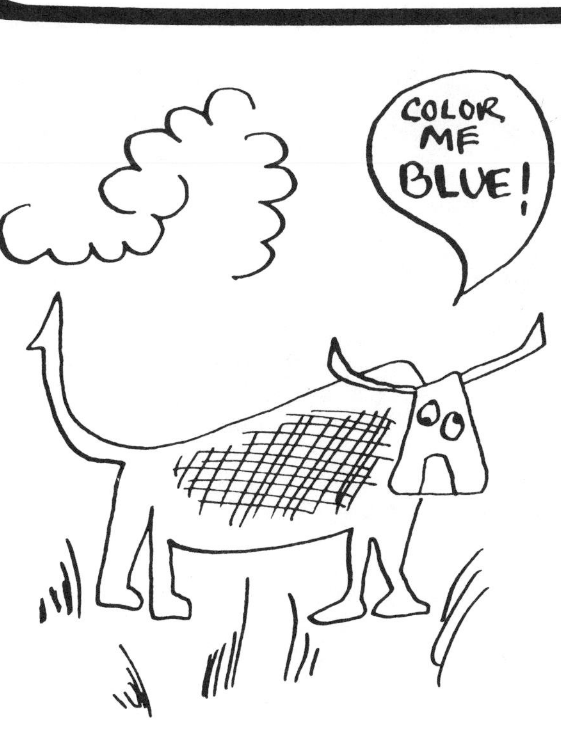

Cyano-

sy-ann-o

blue appearance of
skin (due to anoxia)

My ox named **Syanno**
has **blue skin**.

A20

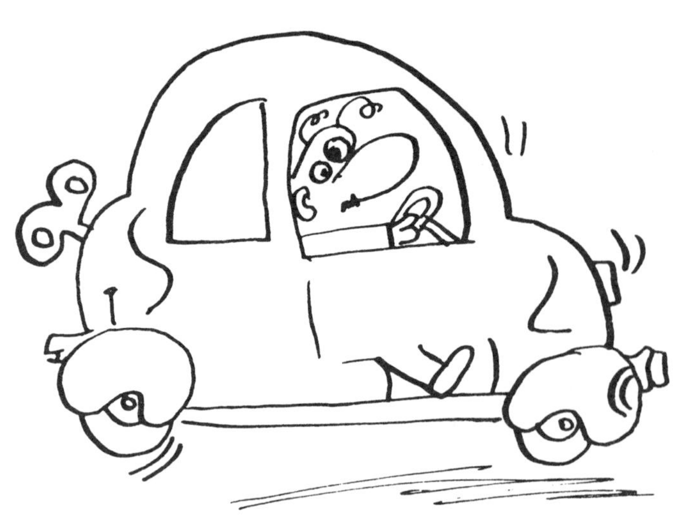

De-

dee

slow down; decrease

Dee power of the car is **slowed down**
by putting your foot on the brake.

A21

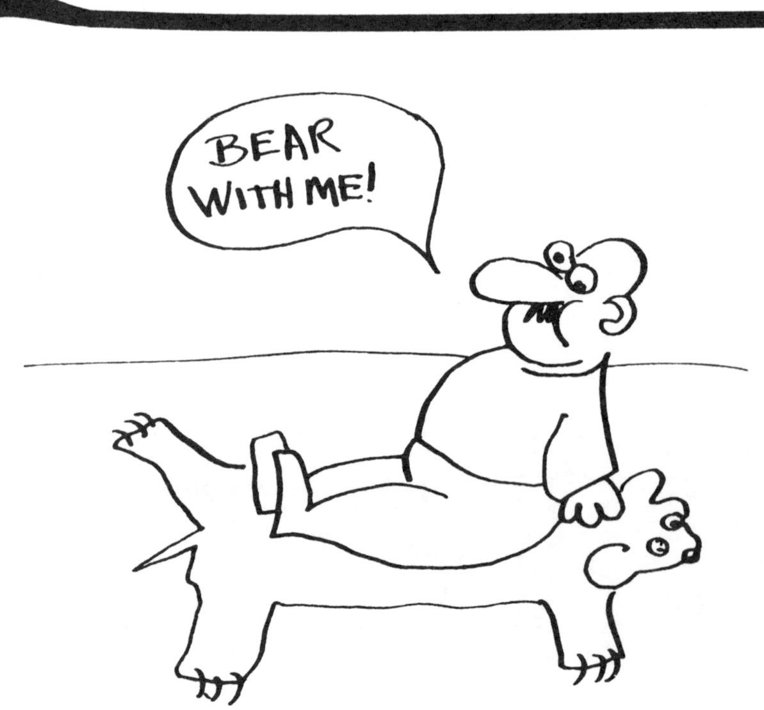

Dermat-

der-maht

skin

Der mott you are sitting
on is made of bear **skin**.

A22

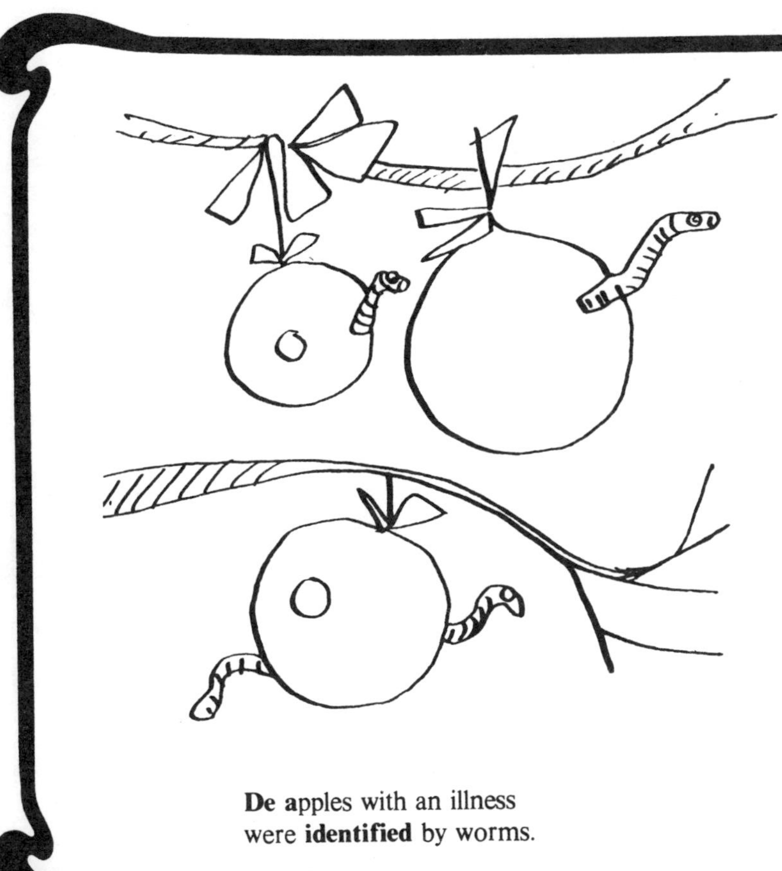

Dia-

dye-a

identification

De apples with an illness
were **identified** by worms.

A23

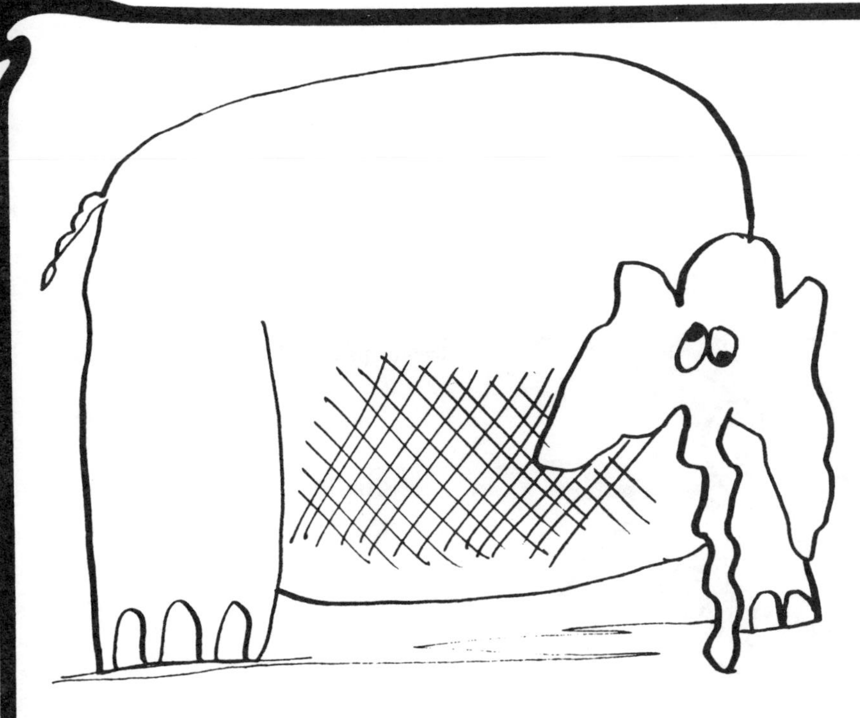

Dist-

dist

part of limb
furthest from trunk

Dis elephant's foot is
far from his **trunk.**

A24

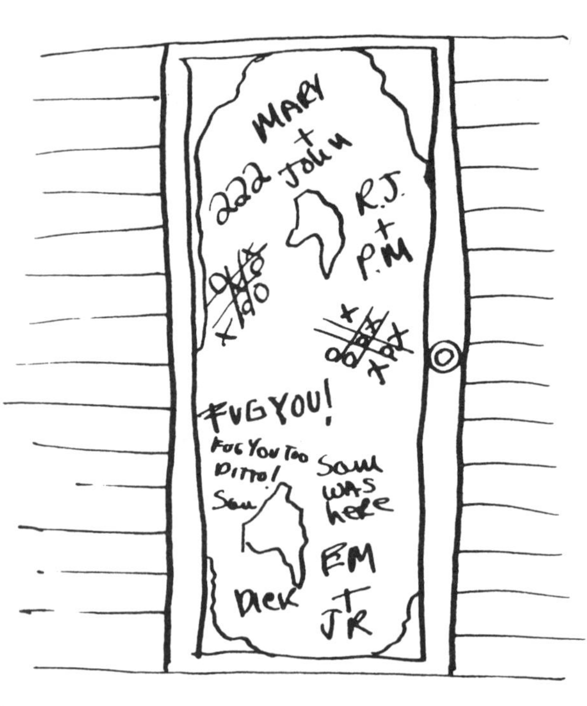

Dors-

dors

back surface of body

The door's back surface
was badly in need of paint.

A25

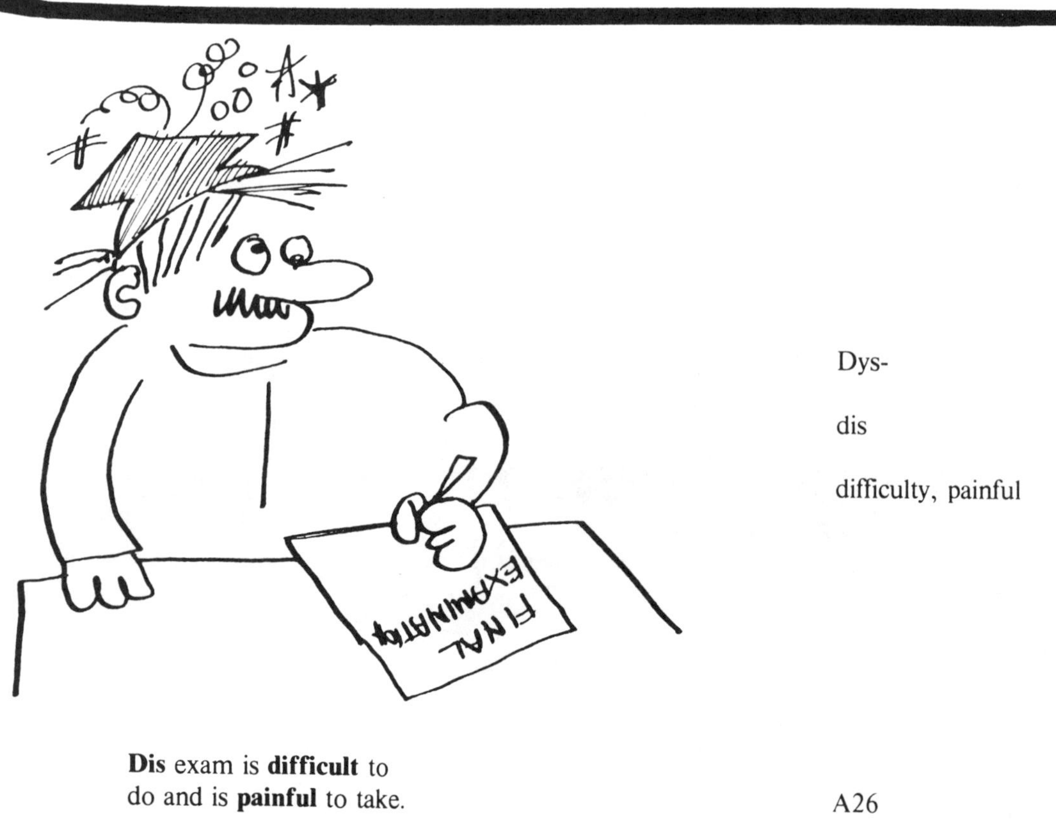

Dys-

dis

difficulty, painful

Dis exam is **difficult** to
do and is **painful** to take.

A26

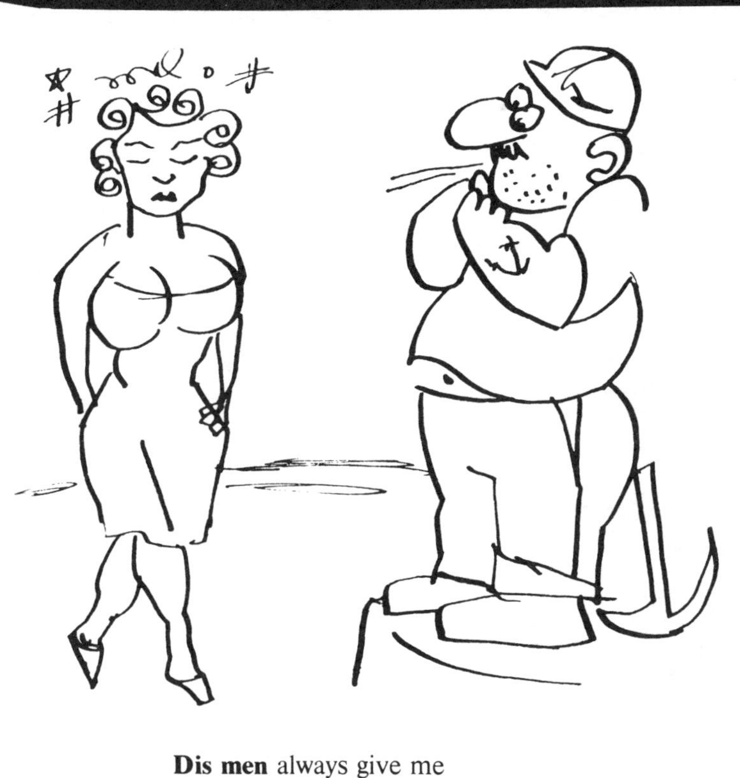

Dysmen-

dis-men

painful menses

Dis men always give me
painful senses in my head.

A27

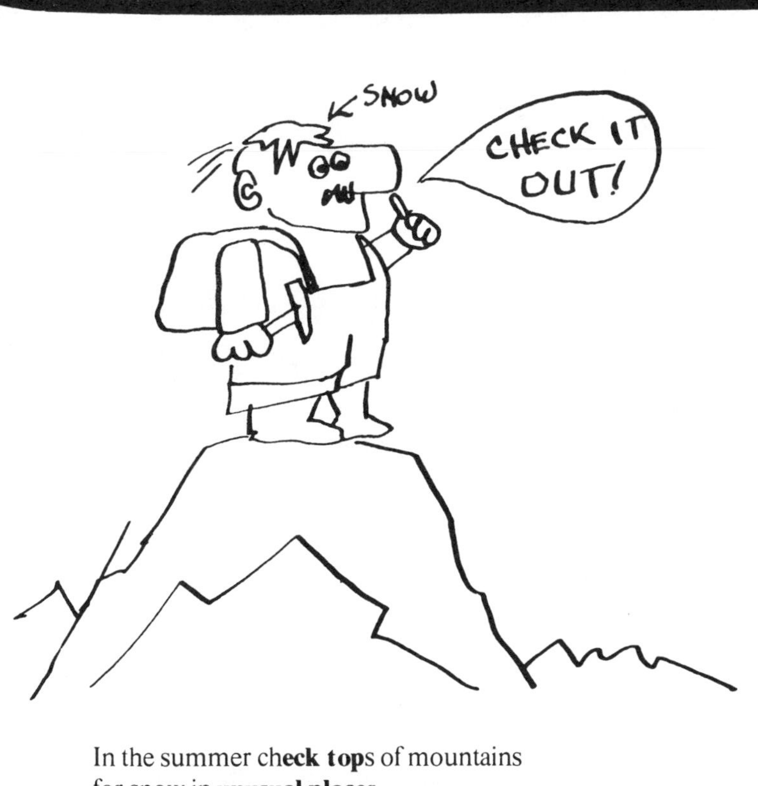

Ectop-

eck-top

to occur outside or
in an unusual place

In the summer ch**eck top**s of mountains
for snow in **unusual places.**

A28

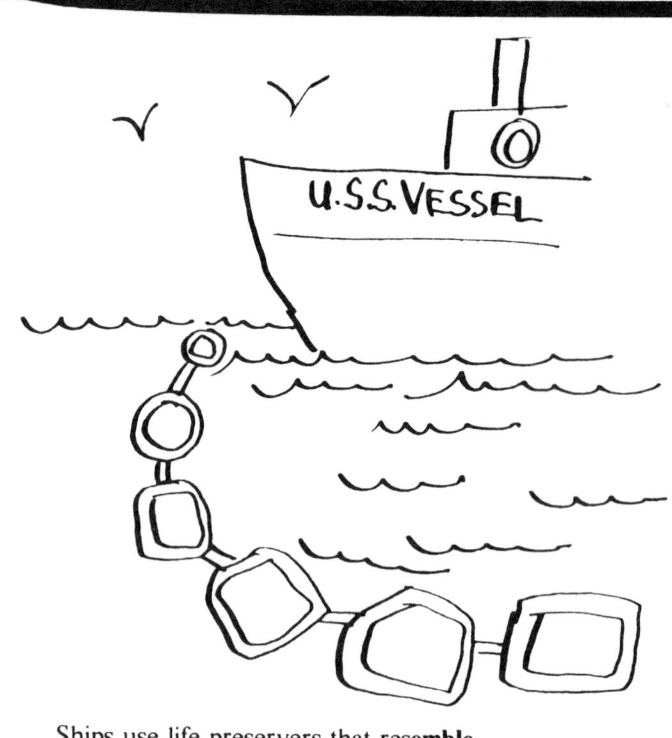

Embol-

em-bol

floating blood clot
blocking vessel

Ships use life preservers that res**emble**
floating lockets for passengers who
must abandon the **vessel**.

A29

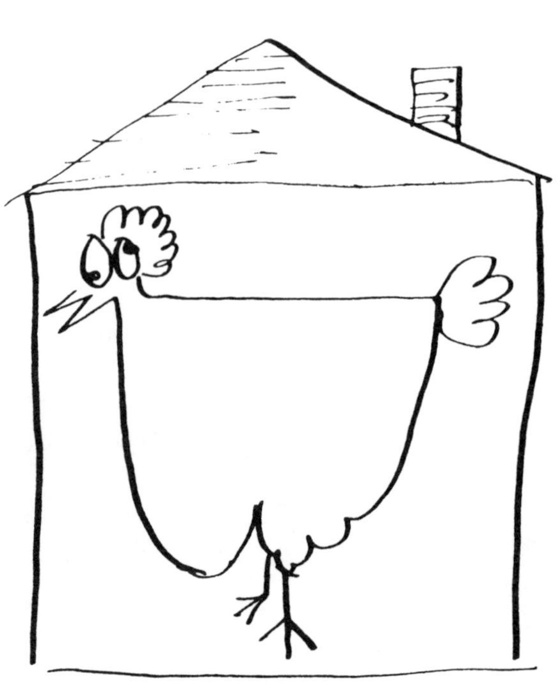

En-

en

inside

Put the h**en inside**
the house.

A30

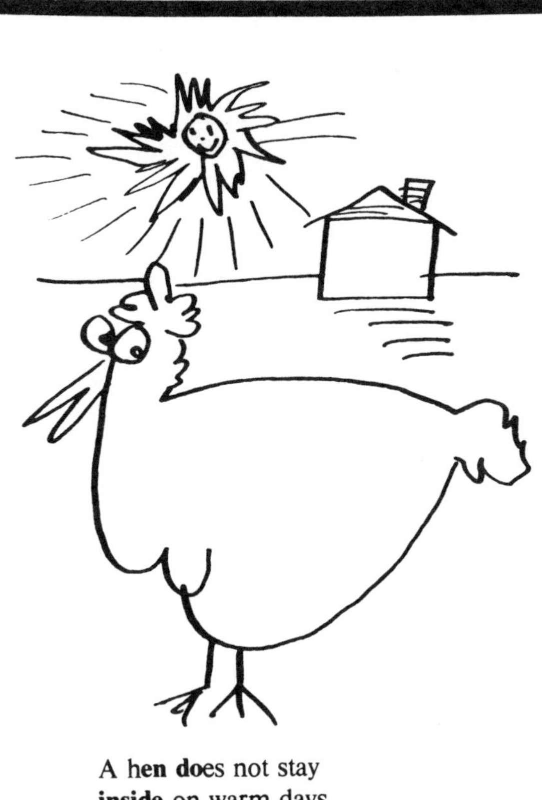

Endo-

en-do

inside

A **hen do**es not stay
inside on warm days.

A31

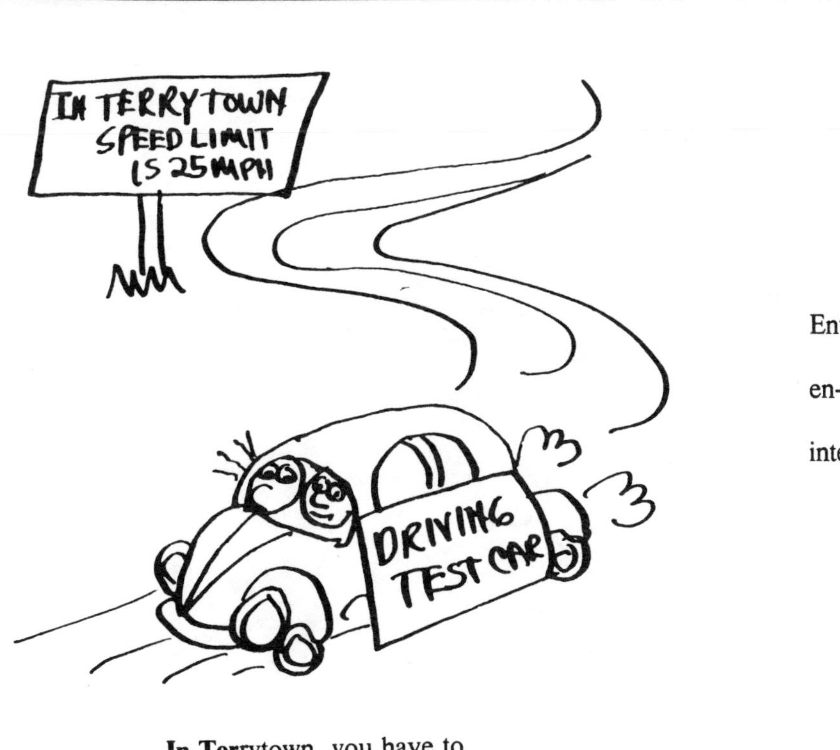

Enter(o)-

en-ter-(o)

intestine

In Terrytown, you have to
take a **test in** driving.

A32

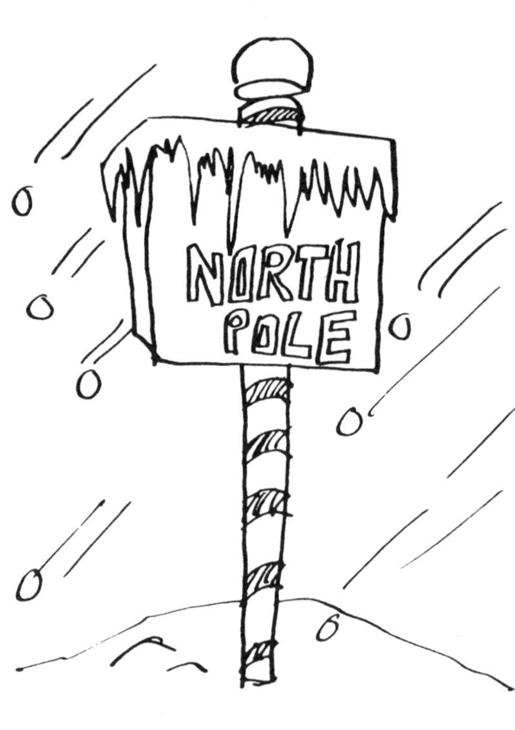

Snow **on top** of the North Pole
is a **normal occurrence**.

Entop-

en-top

occurring in a
normal place

A33

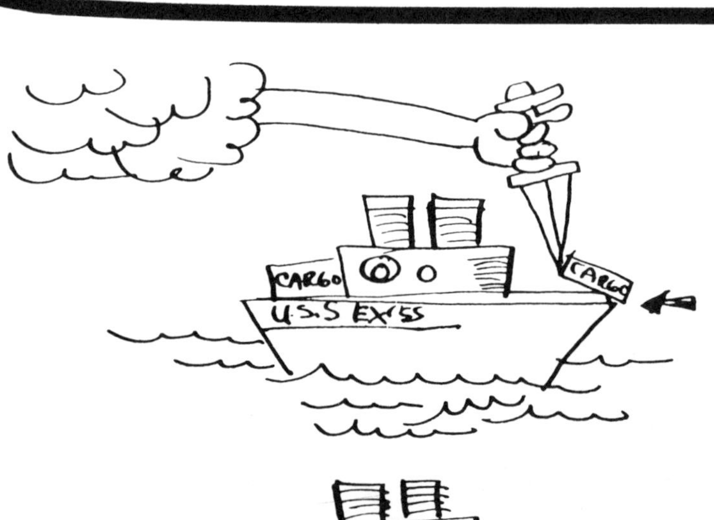

You change the **deck size** of
a ship by **cutting out** cargo.

Excis-

eck-siz

remove by cutting out

A34

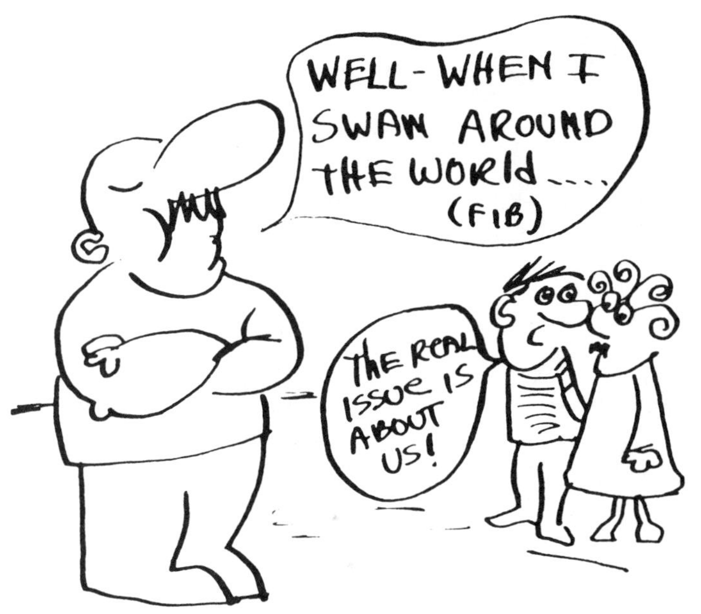

Fibr-

fi-br

fibrous tissue

He always told **fibs**, but the **fib** ab**out us**
is the **issue** we are talking about.

A35

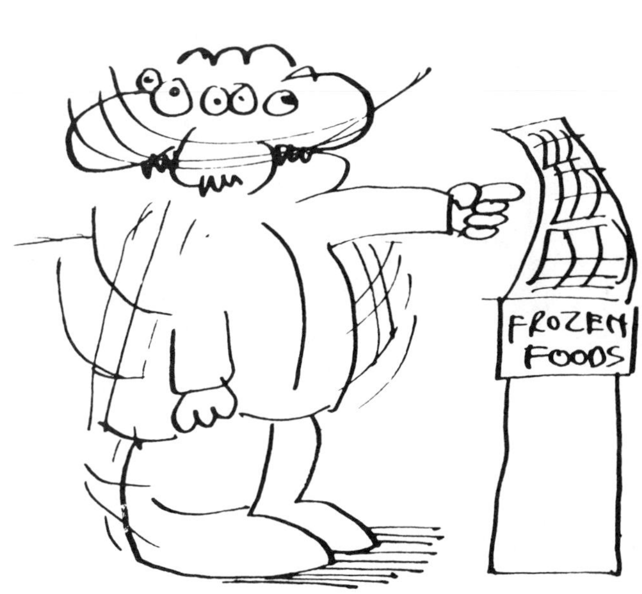

Frozen

fro-zen

rapid examination
of tissue

I looked rapidly at
the **frozen** foods.

A36

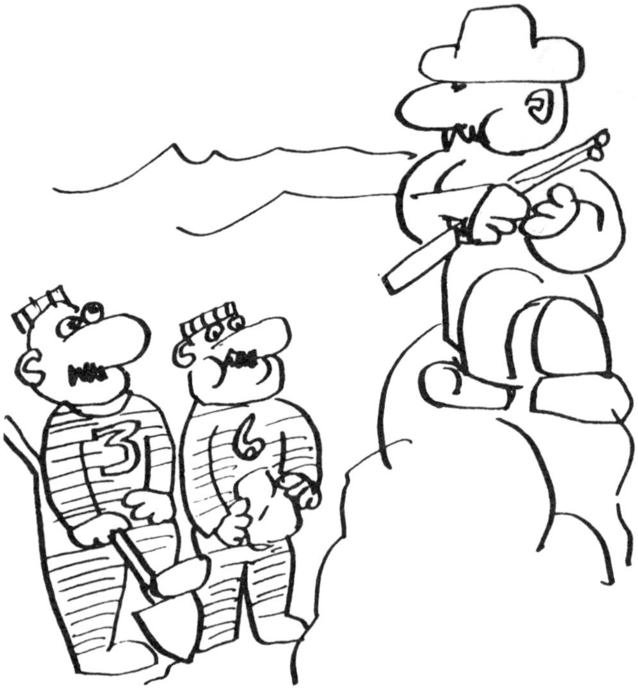

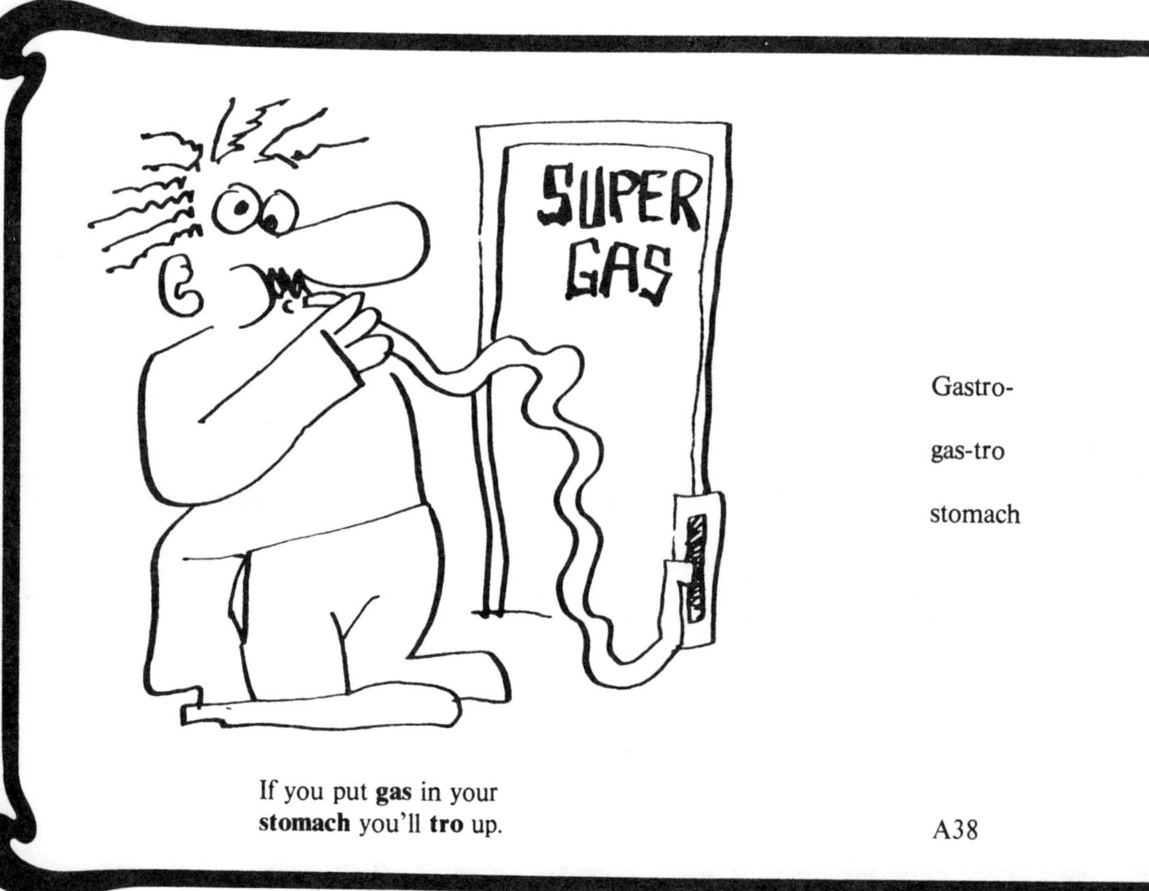

Gall

gaul

bile

It **galls** me that he
sits **bile** we work.

A37

Gastro-

gas-tro

stomach

If you put **gas** in your
stomach you'll **tro** up.

A38

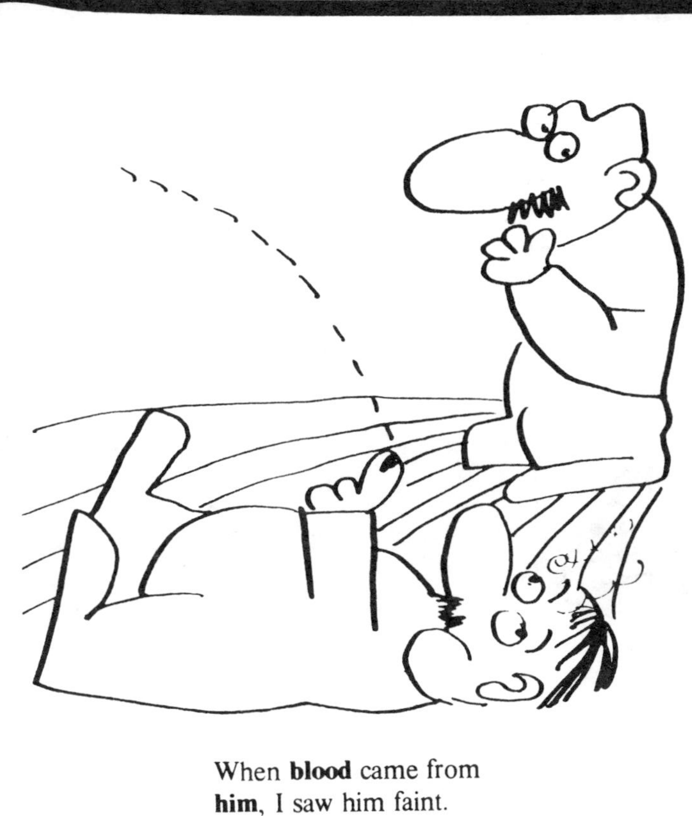

Hem(at)-

hehm-(at)

blood

When **blood** came from
him, I saw him faint.

A39

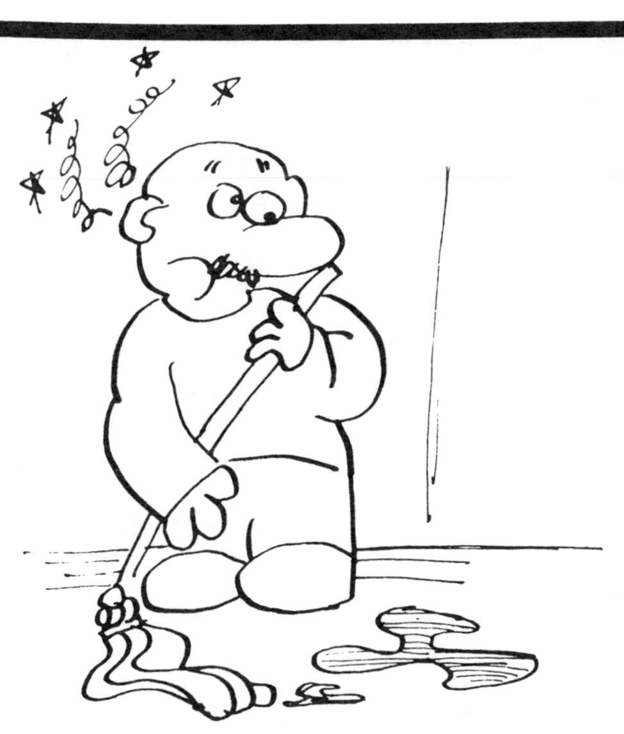

Hemopty-

hee-mop-tah

spit blood from lungs

He mopped up the
blood he **spit** out.

A40

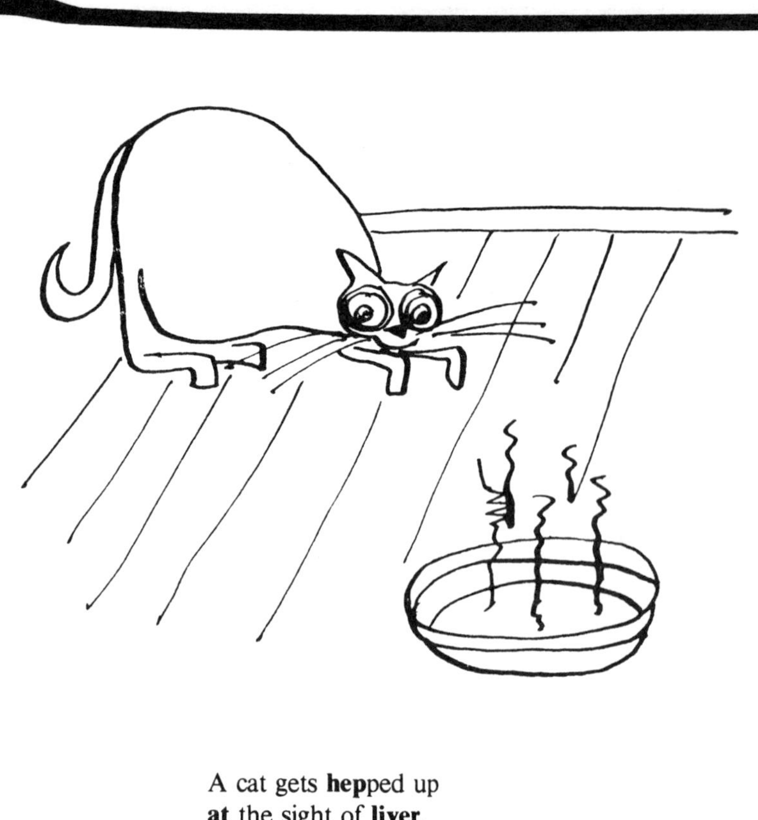

Hepat-

hep-at

liver

A cat gets hepped up
at the sight of **liver**.

A41

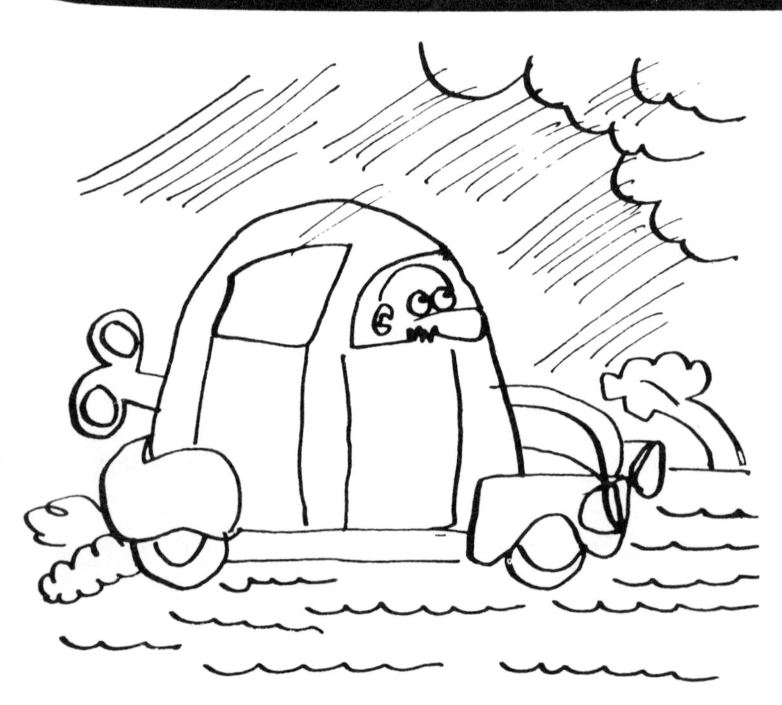

Hydro-

hy-dro

water

Hy drove his car
through **water**.

A42

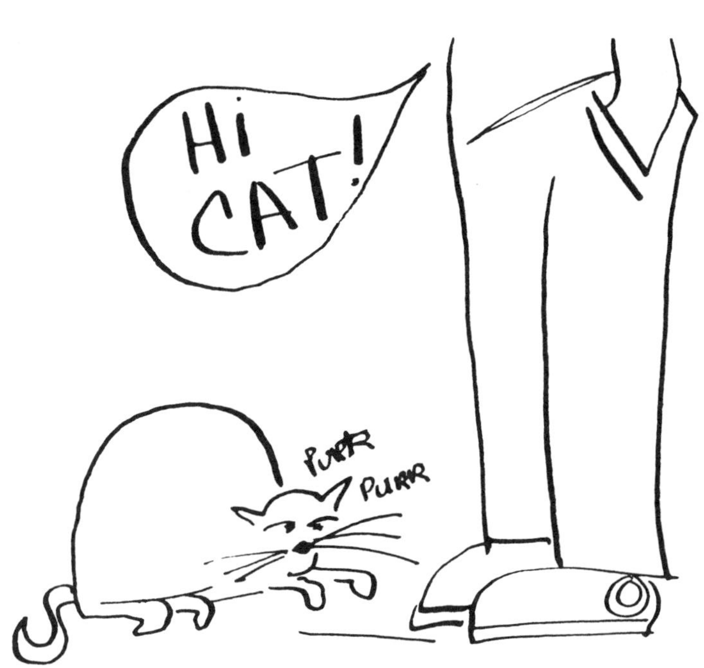

Hyper-

hy-purr

over; excessively

When I said "**Hi,** cat,"he **purr**ed
excessively and came **over.**

A43

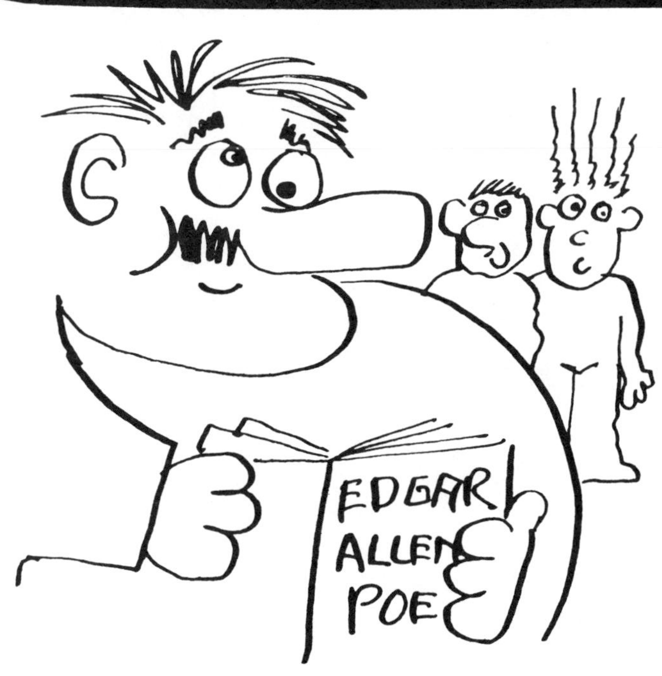

Hystero-

hiss-ter-o

uterus

I was **hysteri**cal when he **us**ed
to **terr**ify **us** with his stories.

A44

WORD/PICTURE ASSOCIATIONS

PREFIXES B

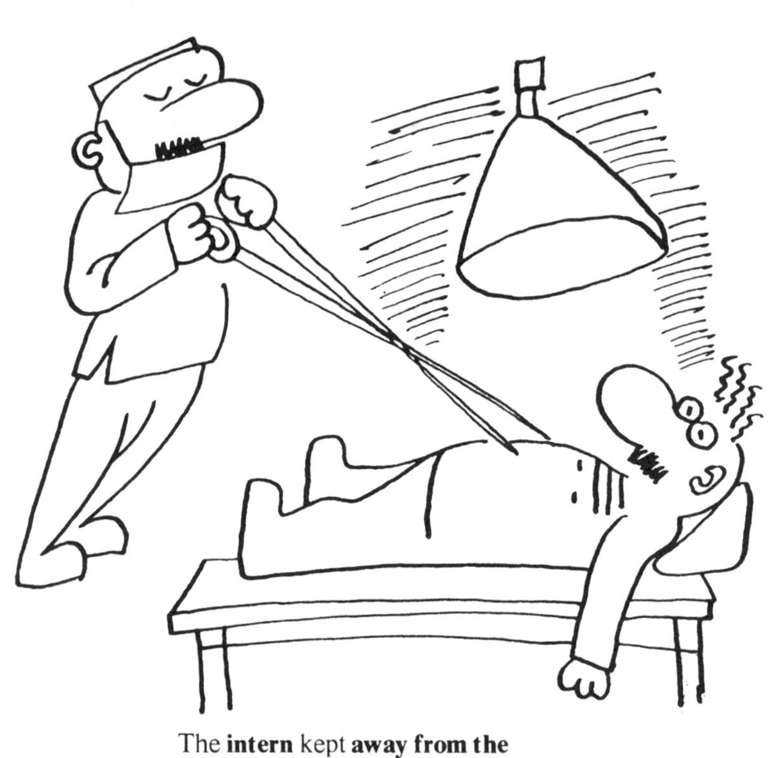

Intern-

in-tern

away from body surface

The **intern** kept **away from the body surface** while cutting it.

B1

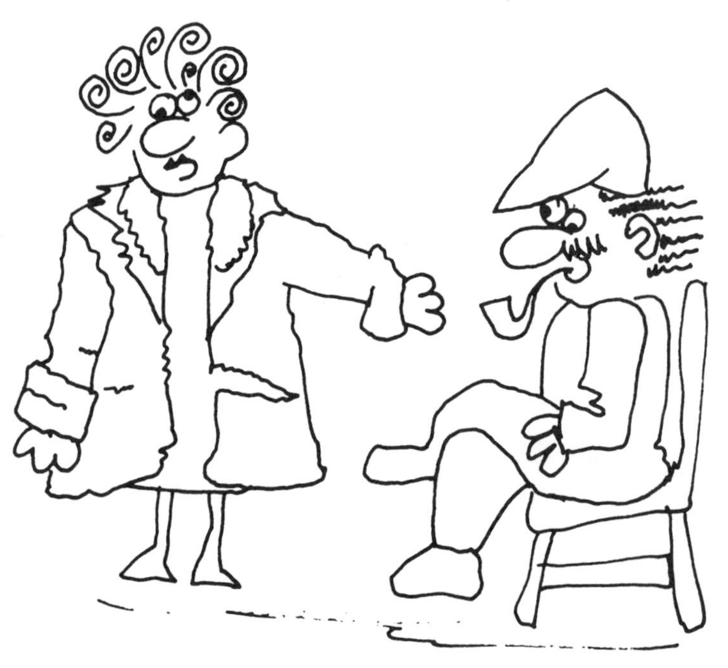

Lacera-

lass-sir-ray

tear or cut in skin

Alas, Sir Ray, I have **torn** the seal**skin** coat.

B2

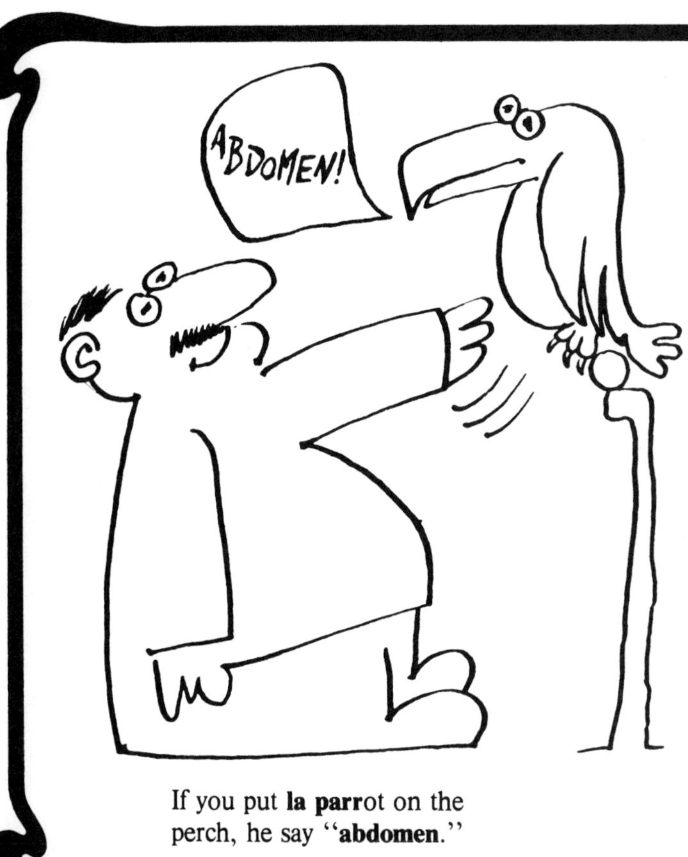

Lapar-

lap-ar

abdomen

If you put **la parr**ot on the
perch, he say "**abdomen**."

B3

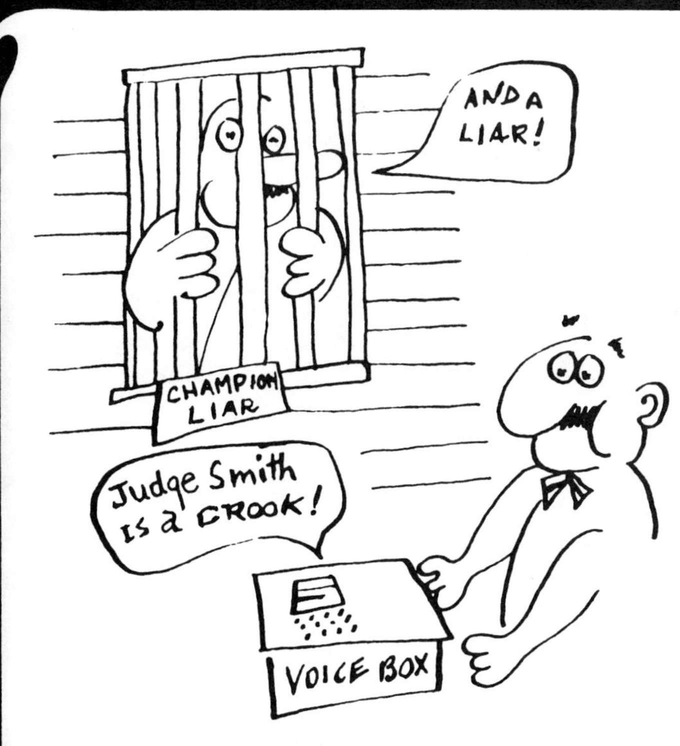

Laryngo-

lar-in-ja

voice box

He put a **lair in ja**il for
saying lies on a **voice box**.

B4

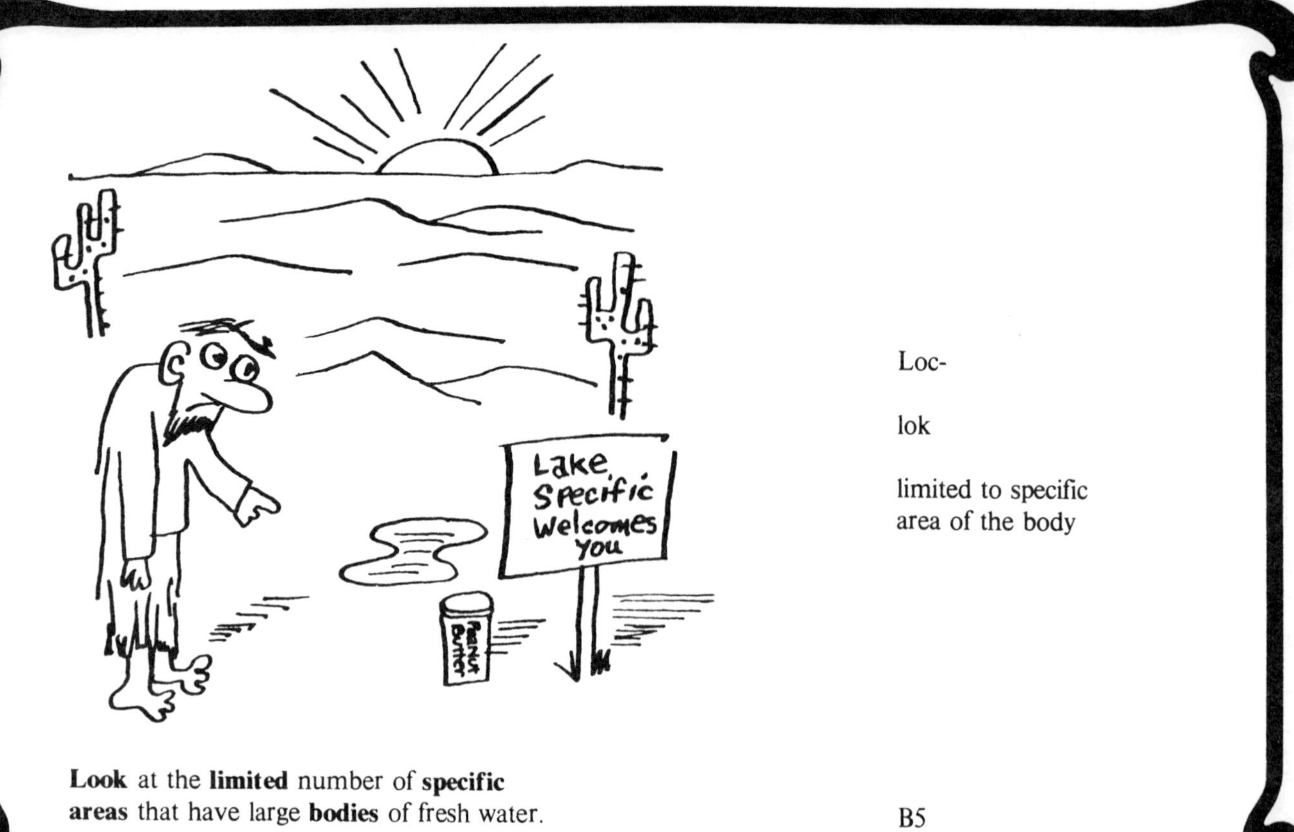

Loc-

lok

limited to specific
area of the body

Look at the **limited** number of **specific
areas** that have large **bodies** of fresh water.

B5

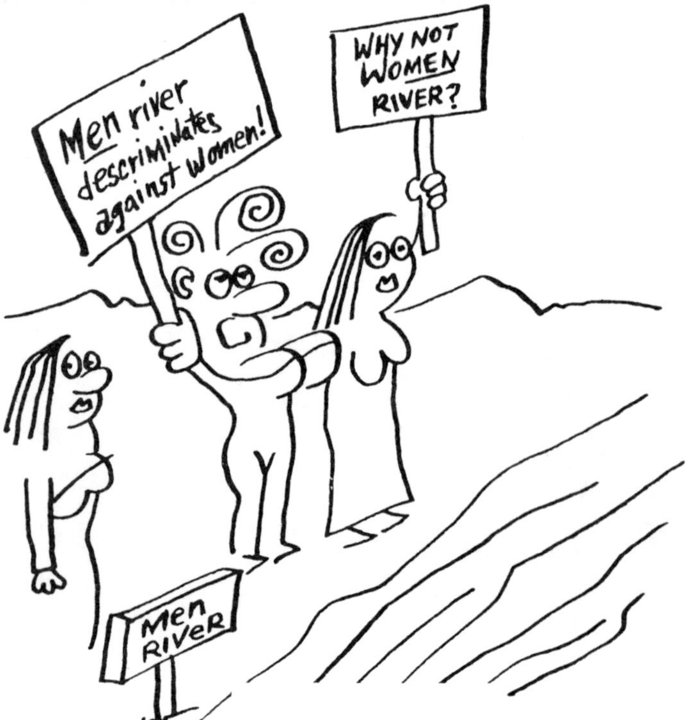

Men-

men

monthly flow

The **Men** River
flows monthly.

B6

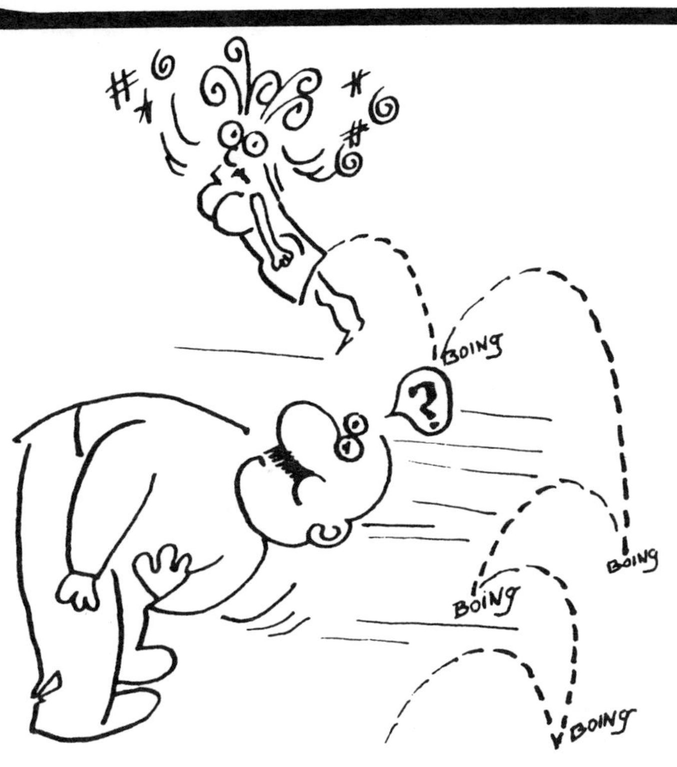

Metasta-

met-tass-tah

disease shifting
from one part of
the body to another

I **met** her and **asked her** to stay but she felt
ill at ease and **moved from place to place**.

B7

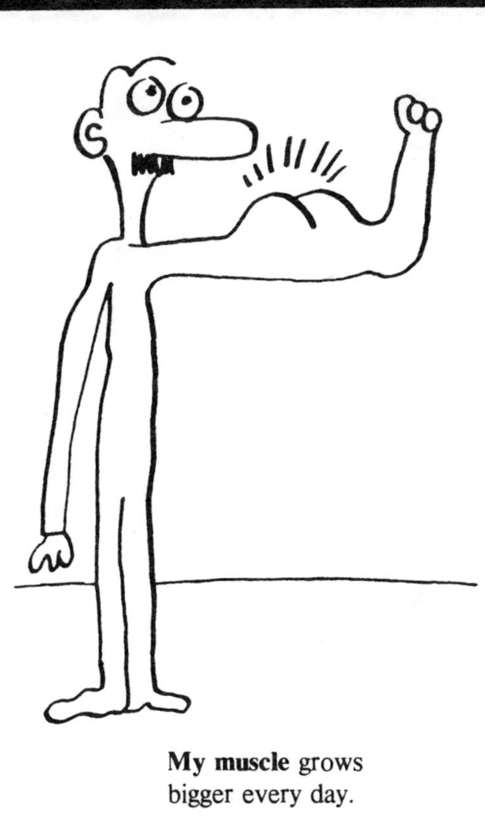

My-

my

muscle

My muscle grows
bigger every day.

B8

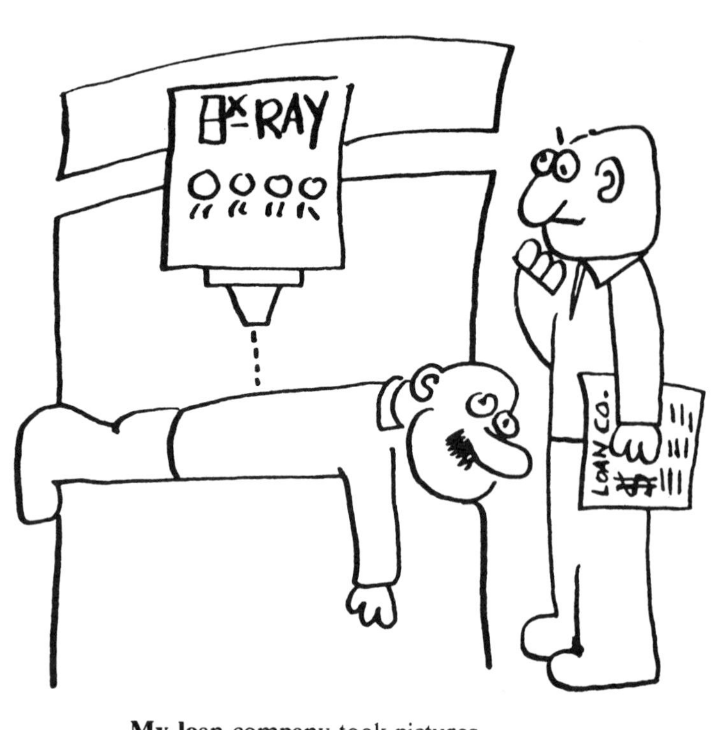

Myelo-

my-lo

spinal cord

My loan company took pictures
of my **spinal cord**.

B9

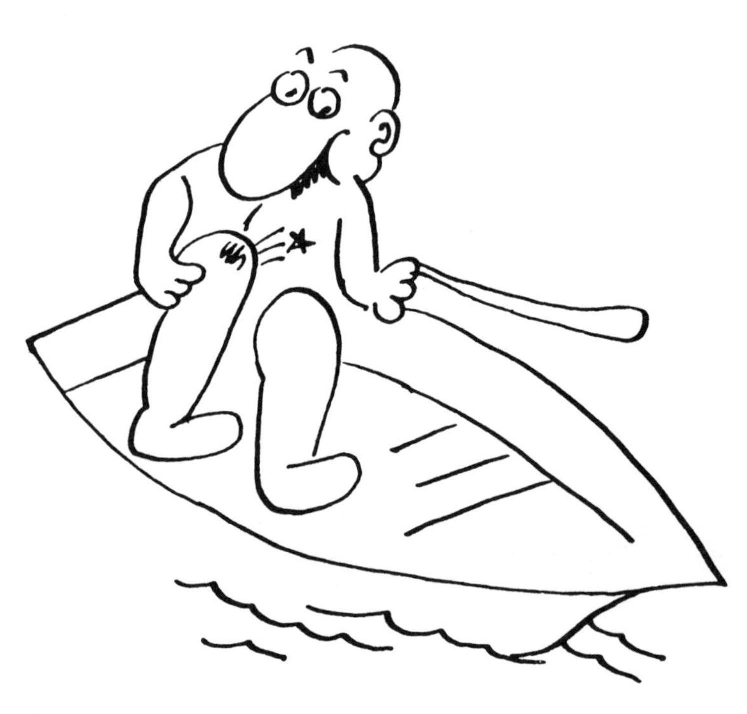

Nephro-

neff-row

kidney

Jeff rowed until he
skinned his **knee**.

B10

Neuro-

new-ro

nerves

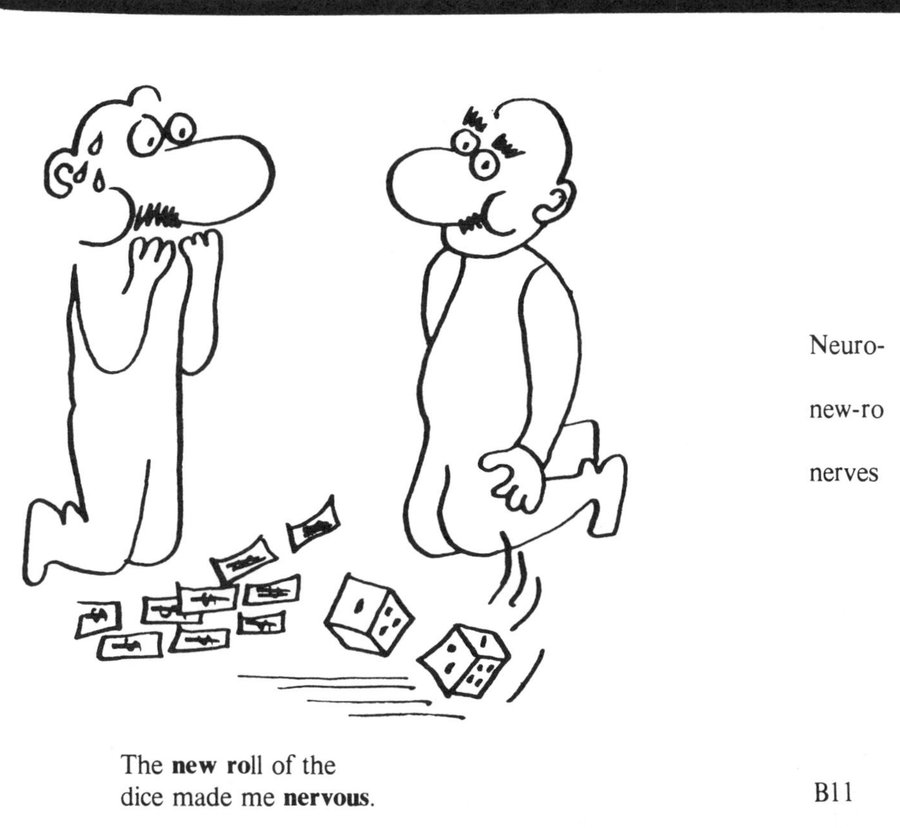

The **new ro**ll of the
dice made me **nervous**.

B11

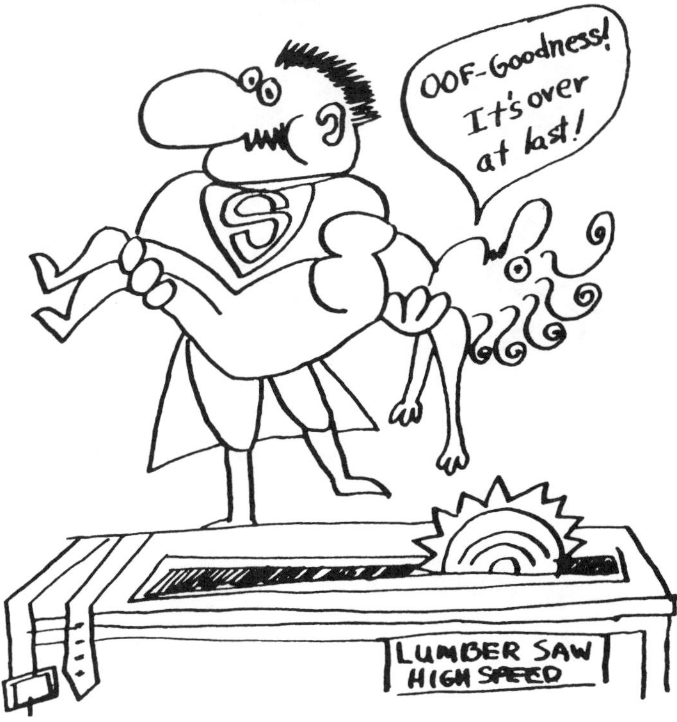

Oophor-

oof-or

ovary

The heroine usually cries "**Oof**!"
or "Goodness, it's **over at** last!"

B12

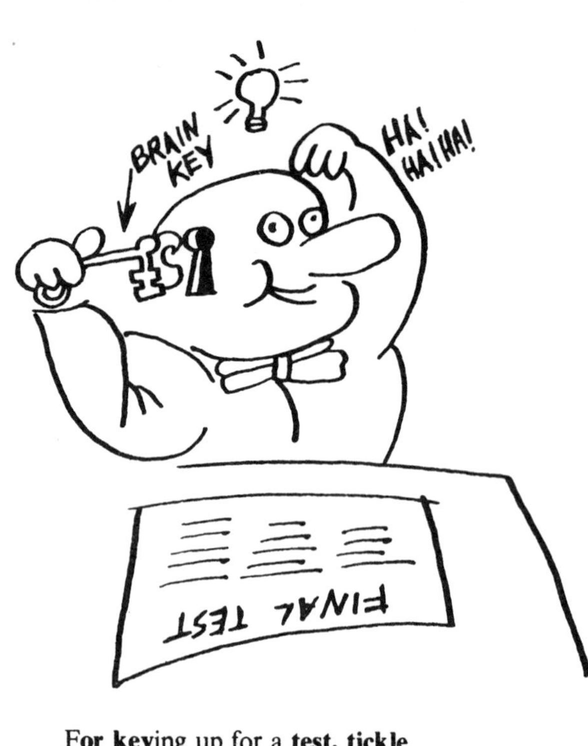

Orchi(do)-

or-key-(do)

testicle

For **key**ing up for a **test, tickle**
your memory and brainpower.

B13

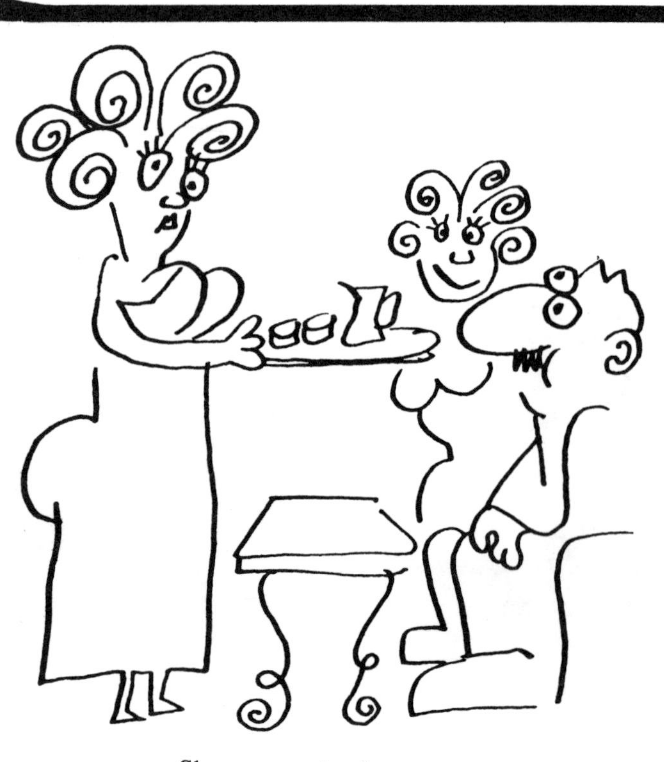

Oste-

oss-tee

bone

She gave **us tea** in
her **bone** china.

B14

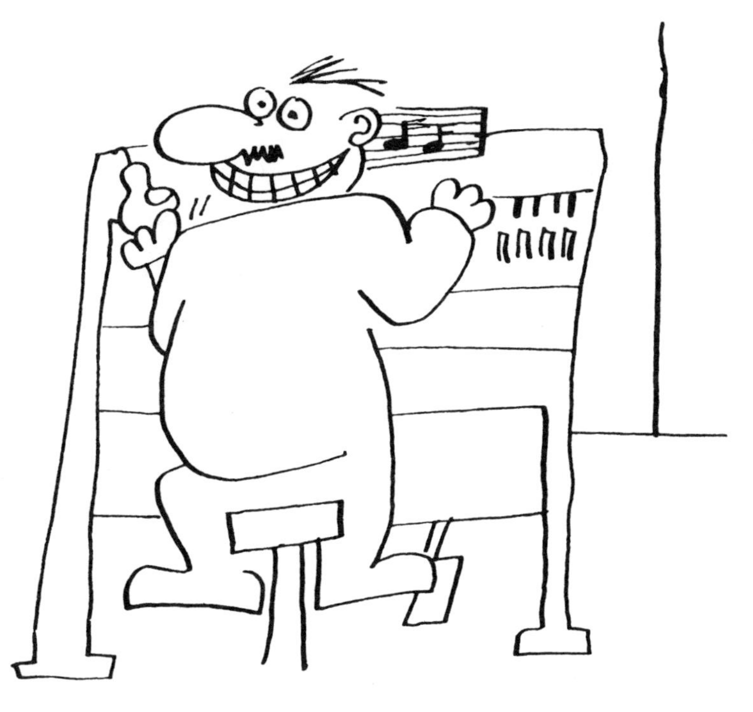

He plays the **organ** while eating a **pear**
and doesn't have **any cavities**.

B15

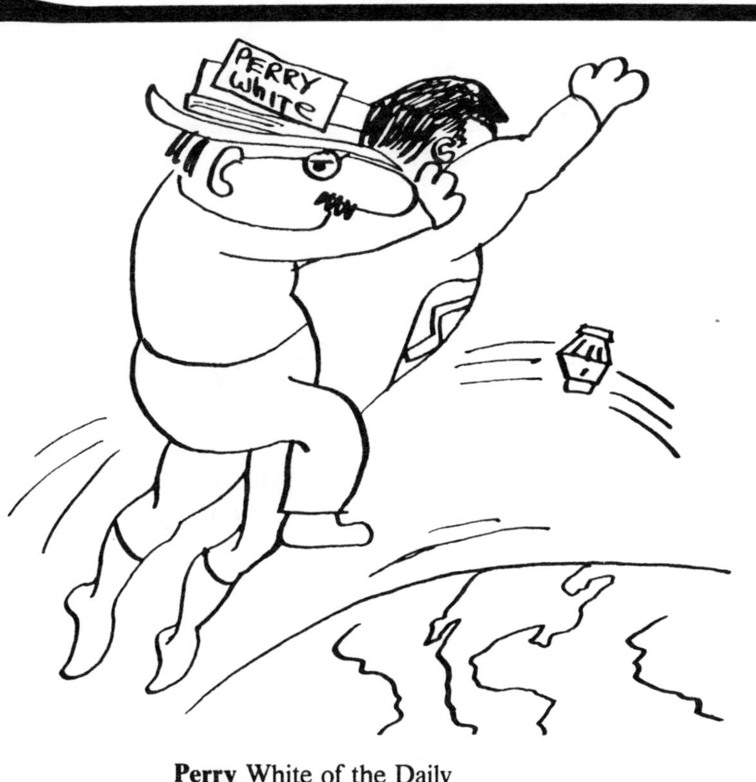

Perry White of the Daily
Planet sure gets **around**.

B16

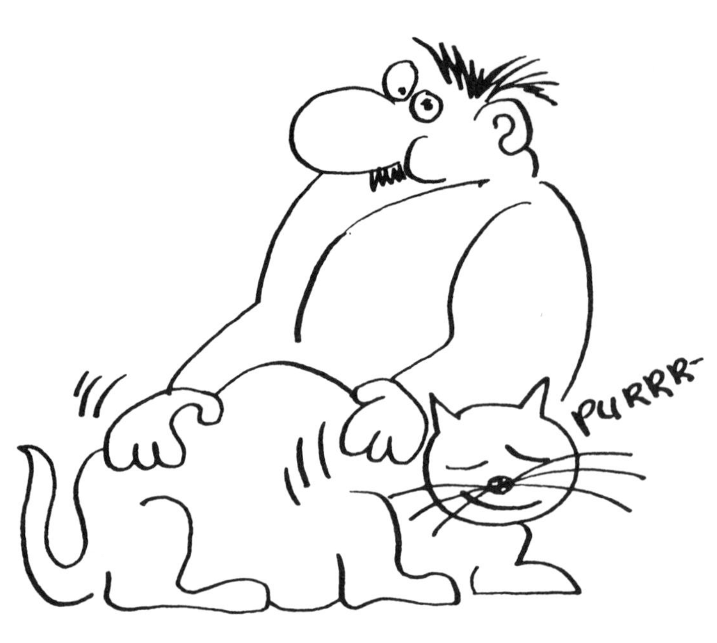

Peripher-

pur-rif-er

outside of; external

The cat will **purr if her outside** fur is petted.

B17

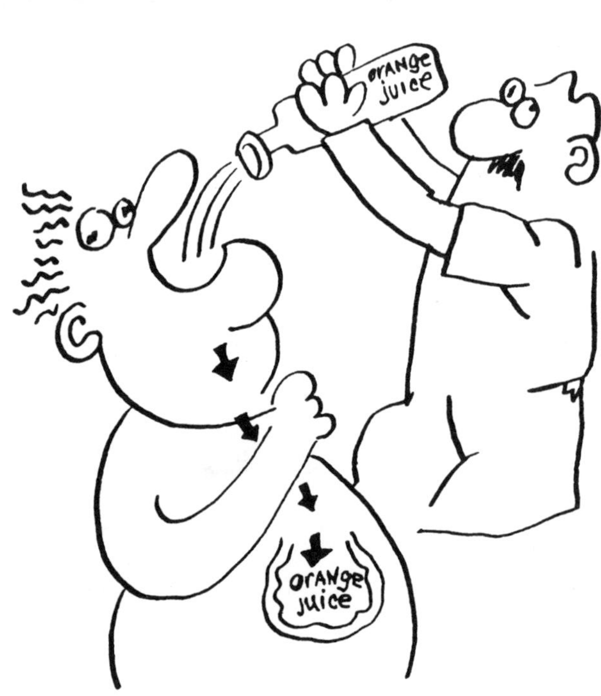

Periton-

per-it-tone

lining inside of
abdomen

Orange juice: **pour it down** the **inside lining of** his **abdomen**.

B18

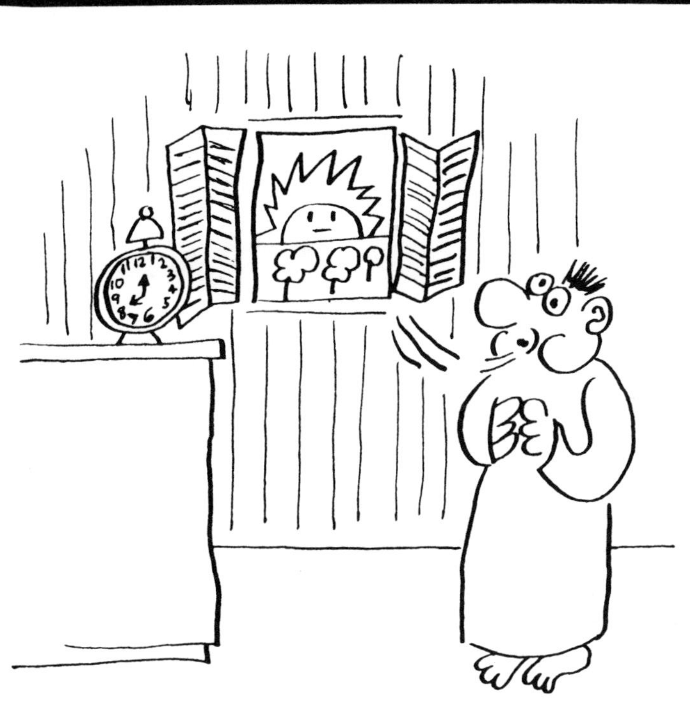

At each **new morn** I
fill my **lungs** with air.

Pneumon-

new-moan

lung

B19

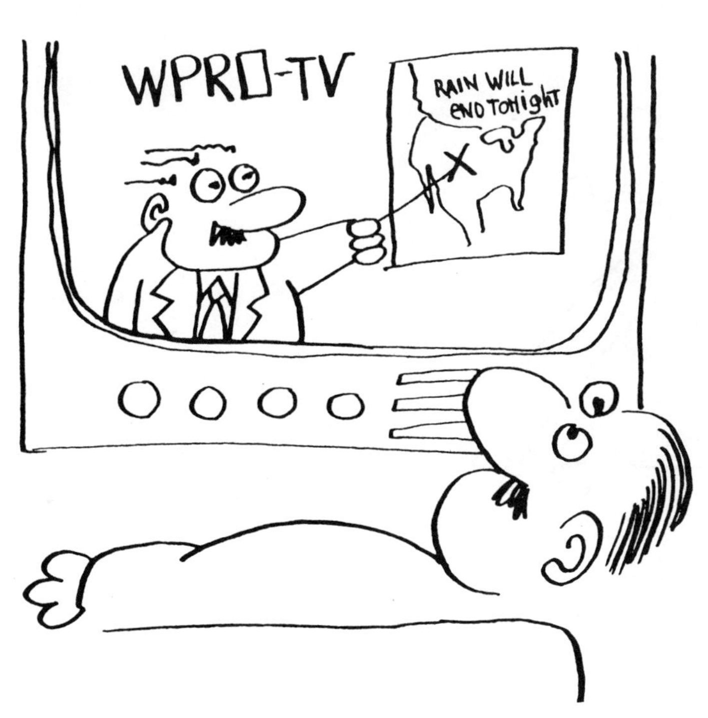

The **pro**gram tells
the weather **forecast.**

Pro-

pro

forecast

B20

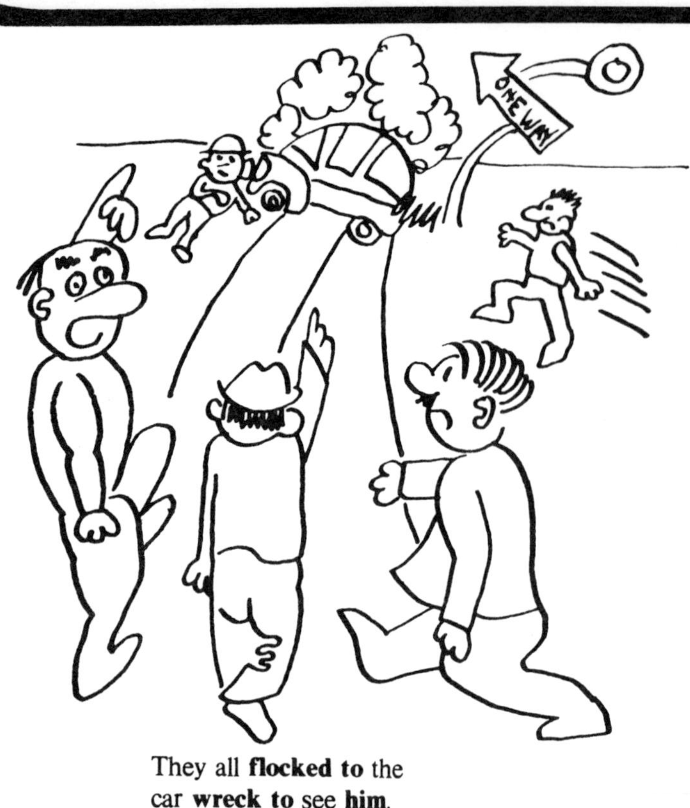

They all **flocked to** the car **wreck to** see **him**.

Procto-

prock-to

rectum

B21

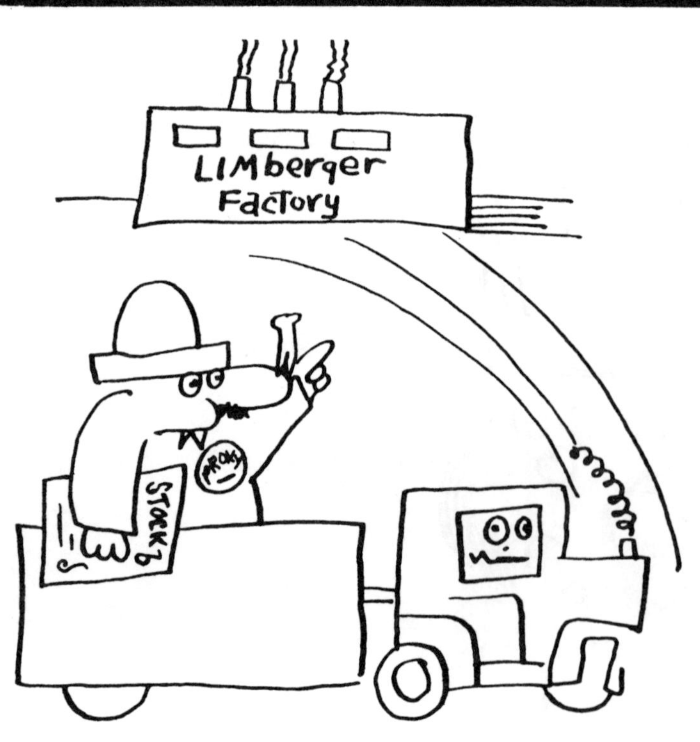

The man sent his stock **proxy** to the **limb**urger cheese factory in a **trunk**.

Proxim-

prox-im

part of limb nearest trunk

B22

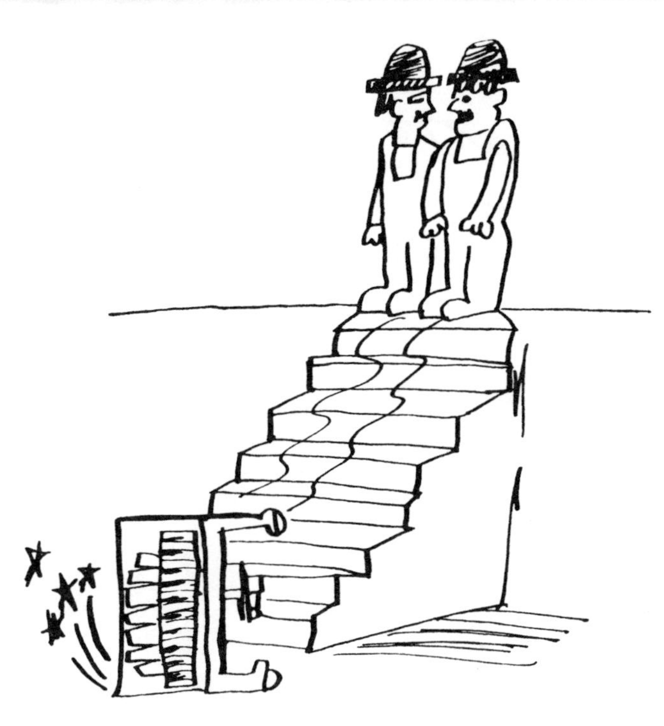

Pto-

tow

drooping of an organ

Tow lines **drooped** when the **organ** fell from the moving men's hands.

B23

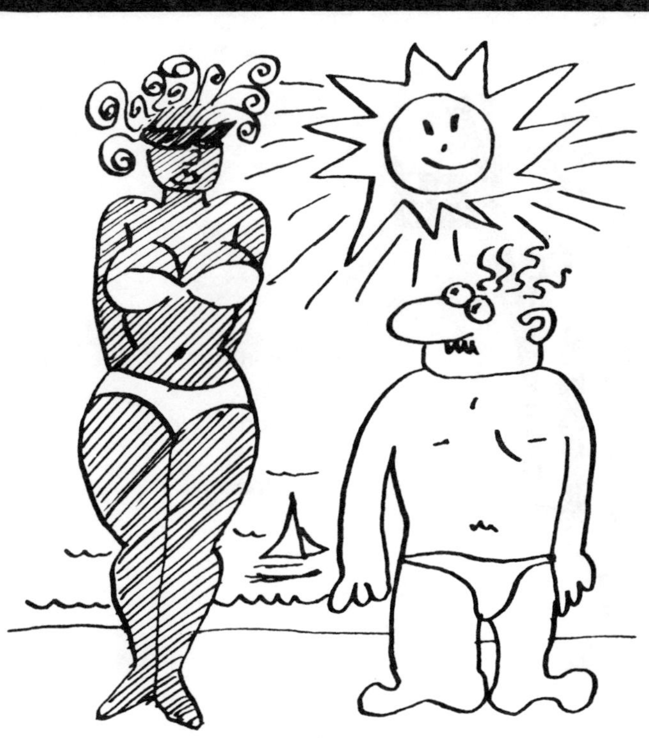

System

siss-tem

entire body

My **sis tem**porarily tans her **entire body** in the summertime.

B24

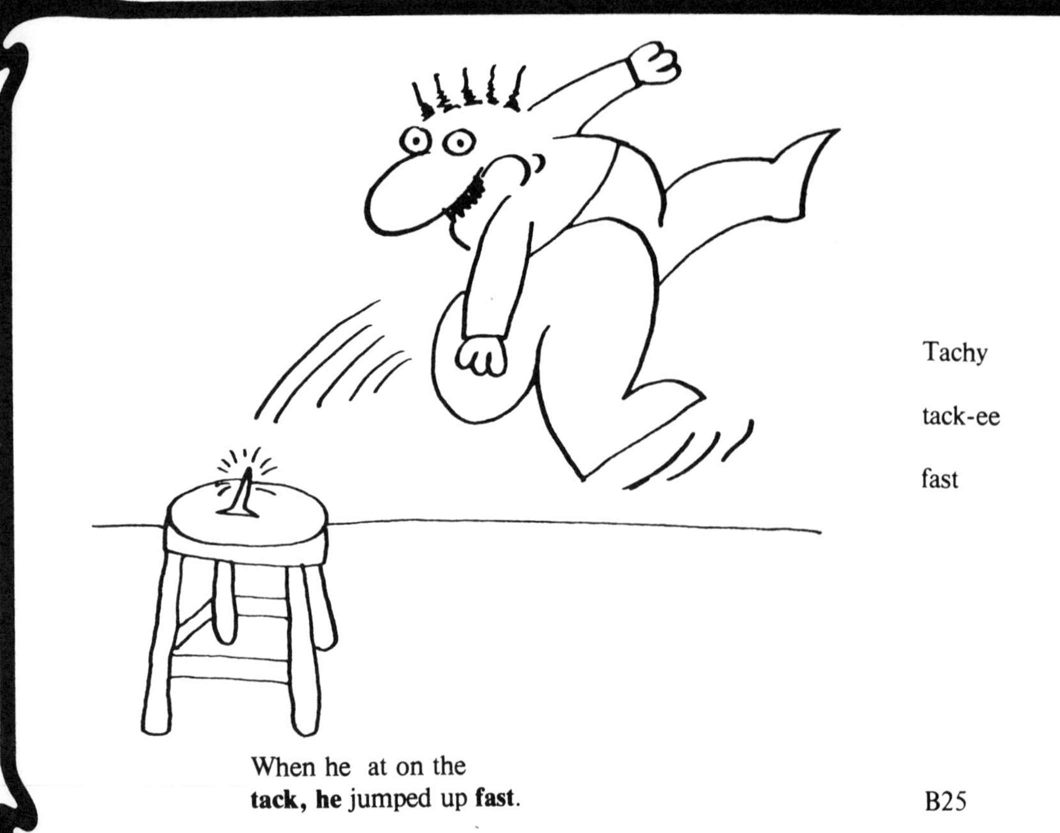

Tachy

tack-ee

fast

When he at on the
tack, he jumped up **fast**.

B25

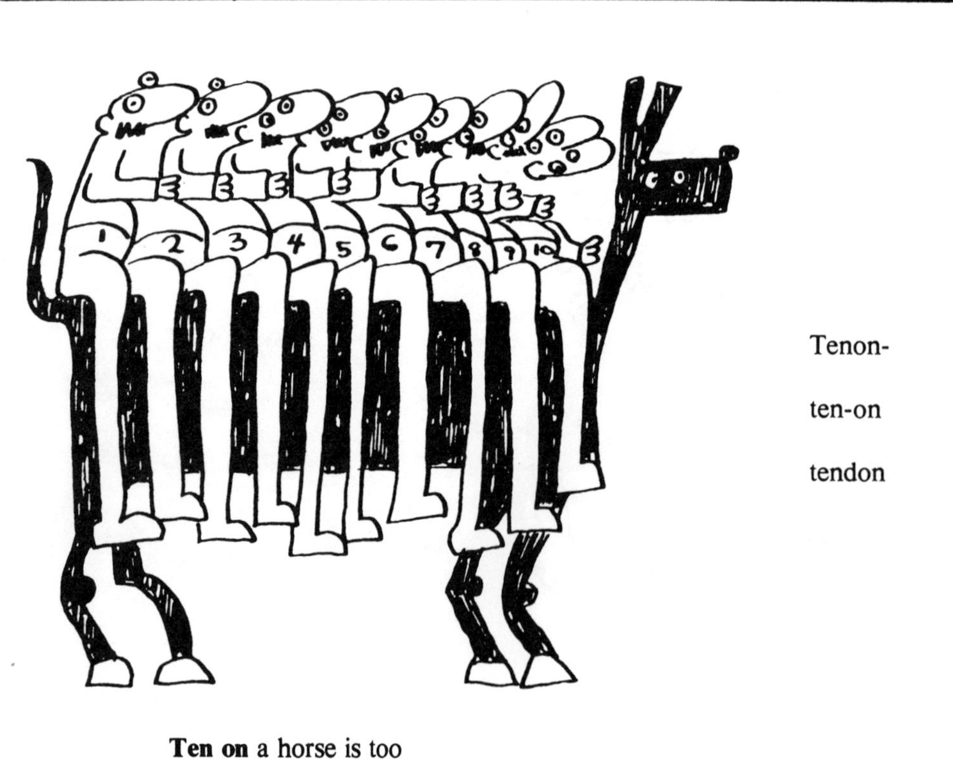

Tenon-

ten-on

tendon

Ten on a horse is too
many to de**pend on**.

B26

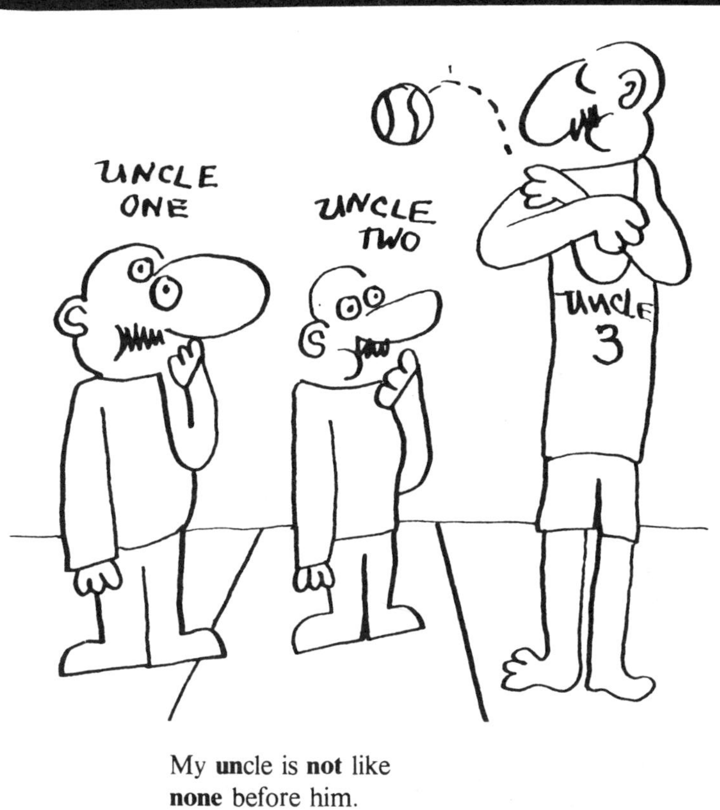

Un-

un

none; not

My **un**cle is **not** like
none before him.

B27

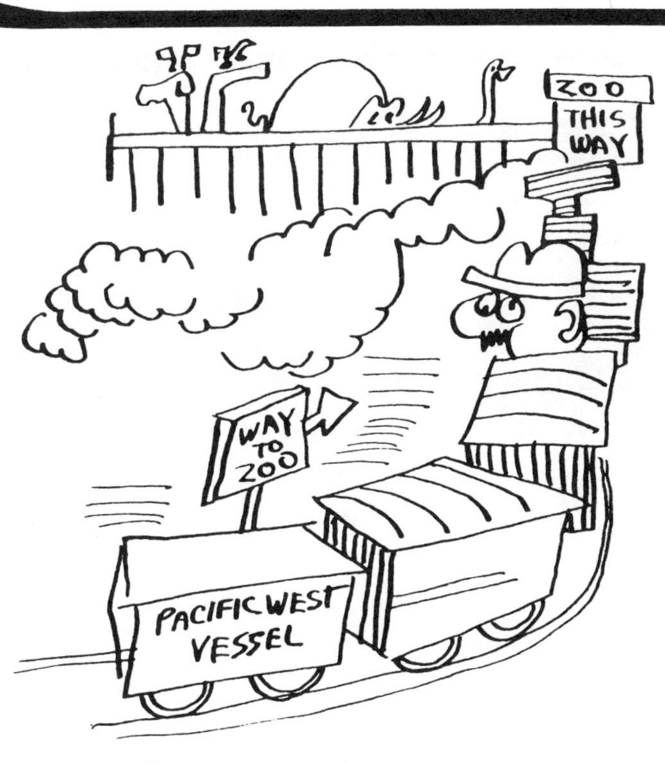

Vaso-

vay-zo

vessel

I went a **way** to the **zoo** on
a **vessel** called a train.

B28

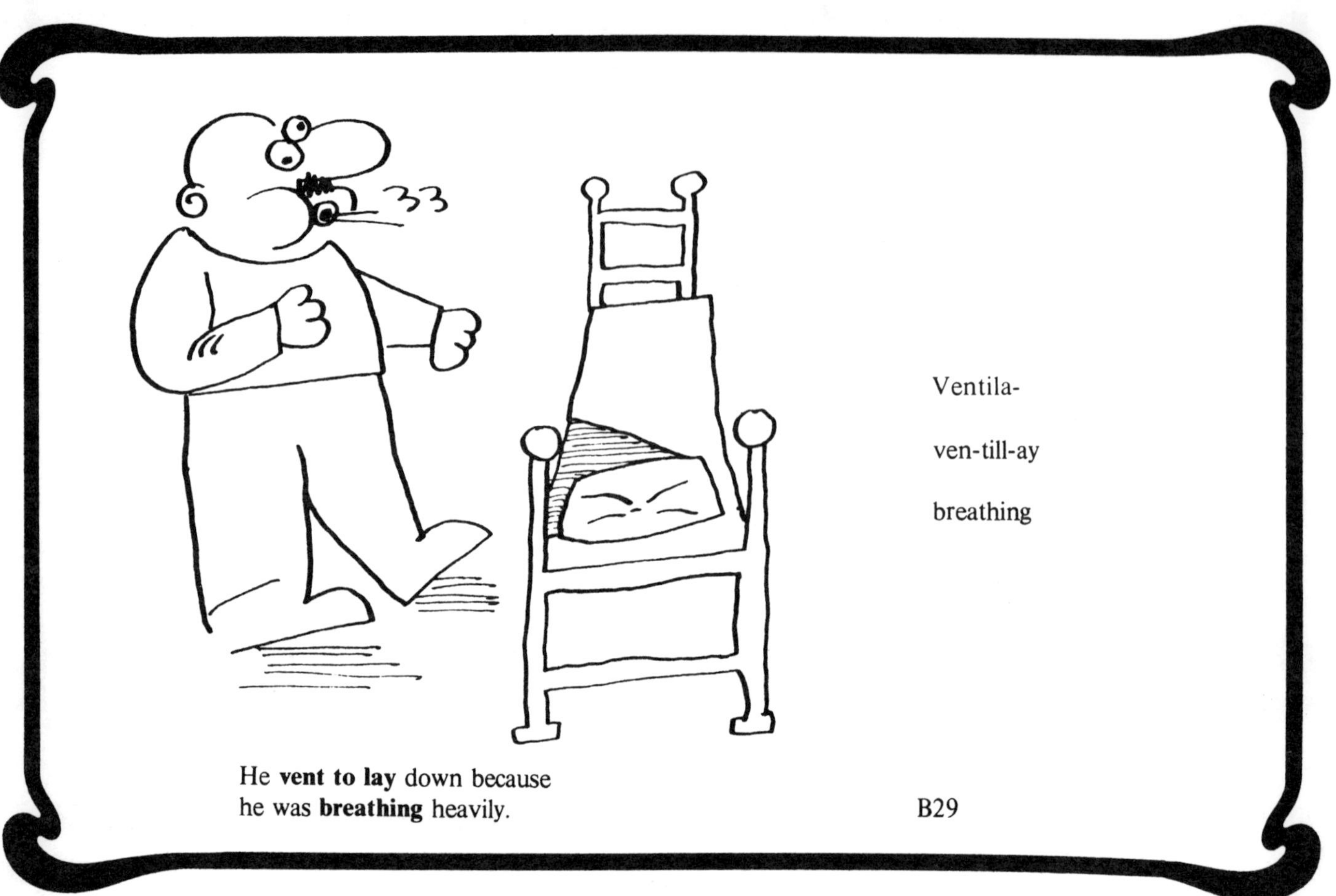

He **vent to lay** down because
he was **breathing** heavily.

B29

WORD/PICTURE ASSOCIATIONS

WHOLE WORDS C

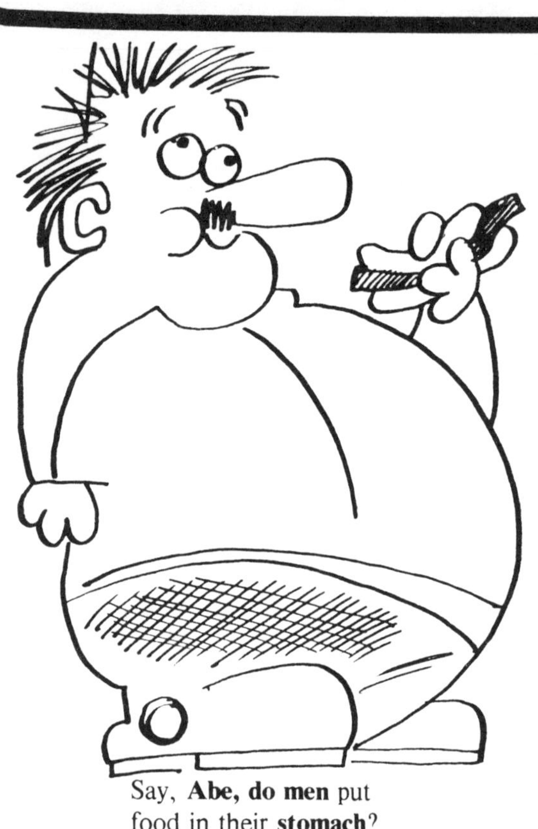

Abdomen

ab-doe-men

stomach

C1

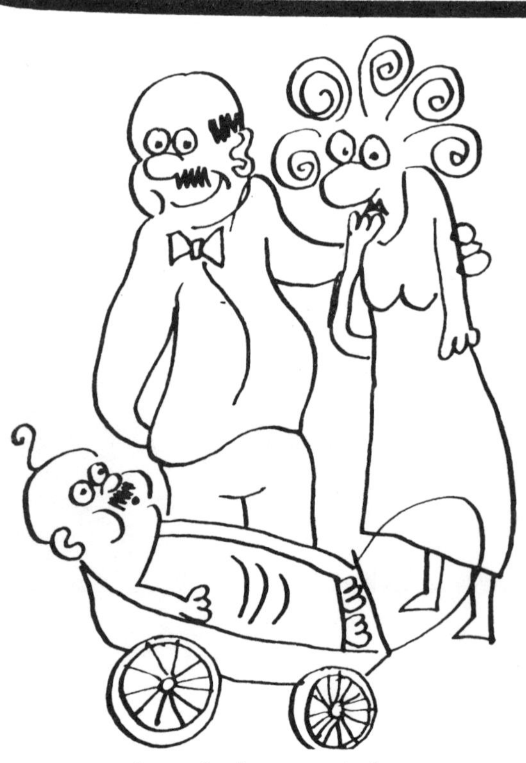

Acquired

ah-quired

developing after birth

C2

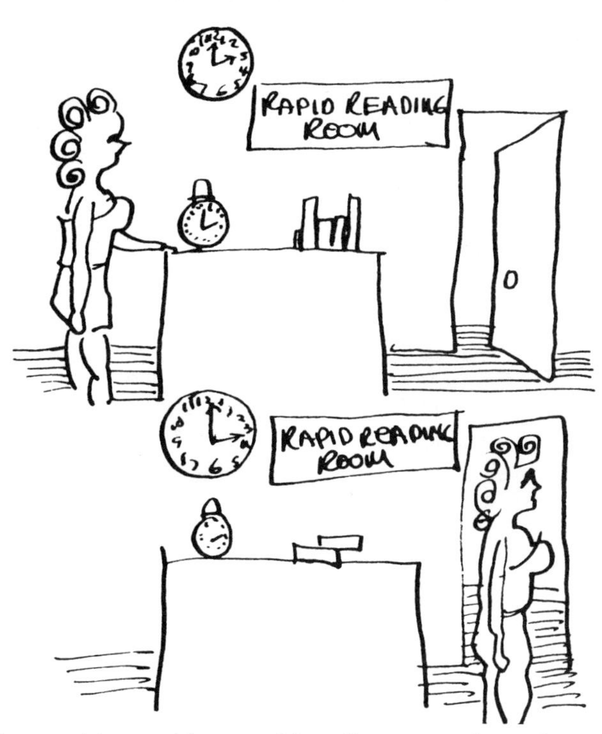

A cute girl was taking a **rapid** reading **course,** but only stayed a **short duration.**

Acute

ah-cute

rapid course;
short duration

C3

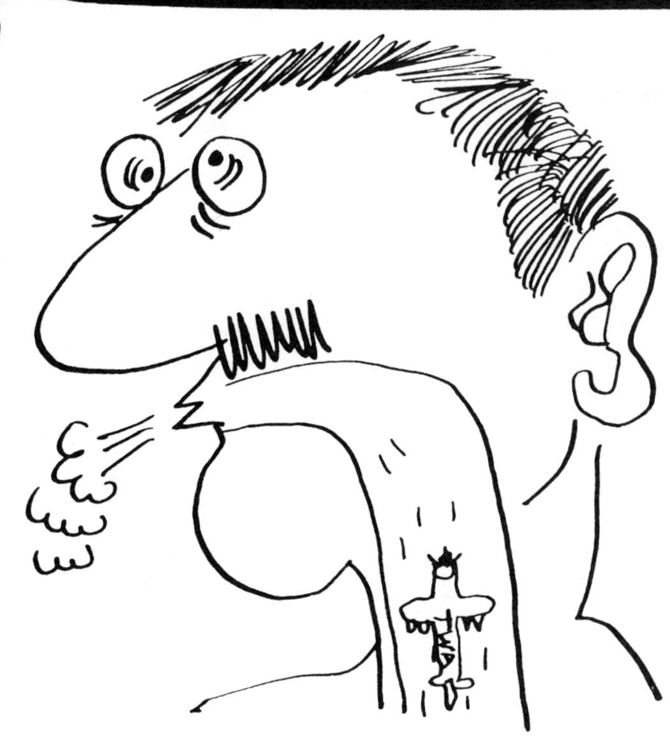

Airway

air-way

entire breathing
passage from mouth
to lungs

Teeny Weeny **Airway** flies the **entire breath-taking passage** for months or longer.

C4

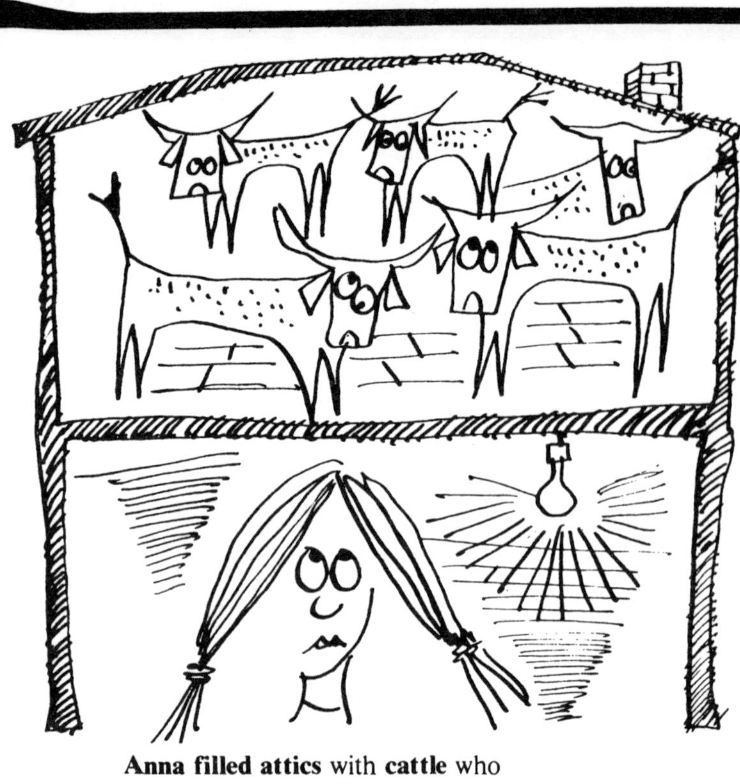

Anna filled attics with **cattle** who **reacted to allergic drugs**.

C5

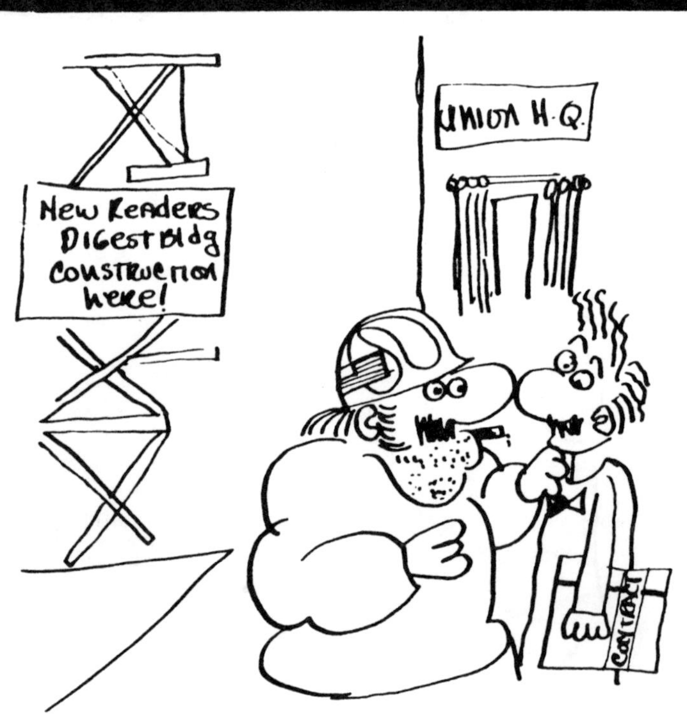

If they don't **pay us** at the **opening** negotiations, in the **end** we'll take the Reader's **Digest** contract!

C6

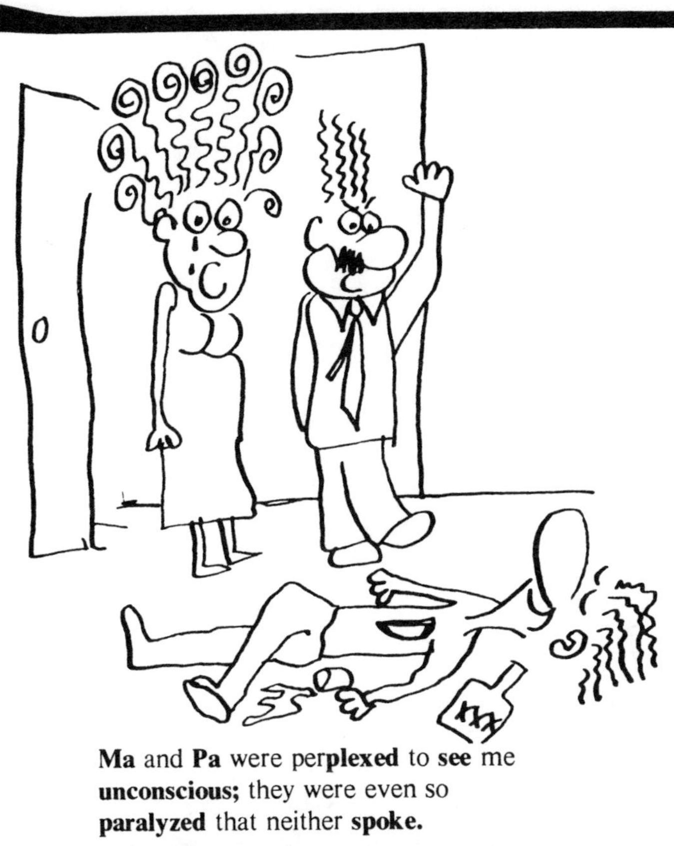

Apoplexy

ah-pa-plex-cee

unconsciousness;
paralysis due to stroke

Ma and **Pa** were per**plexed** to **see** me
unconscious; they were even so
paralyzed that neither **spoke.**

C7

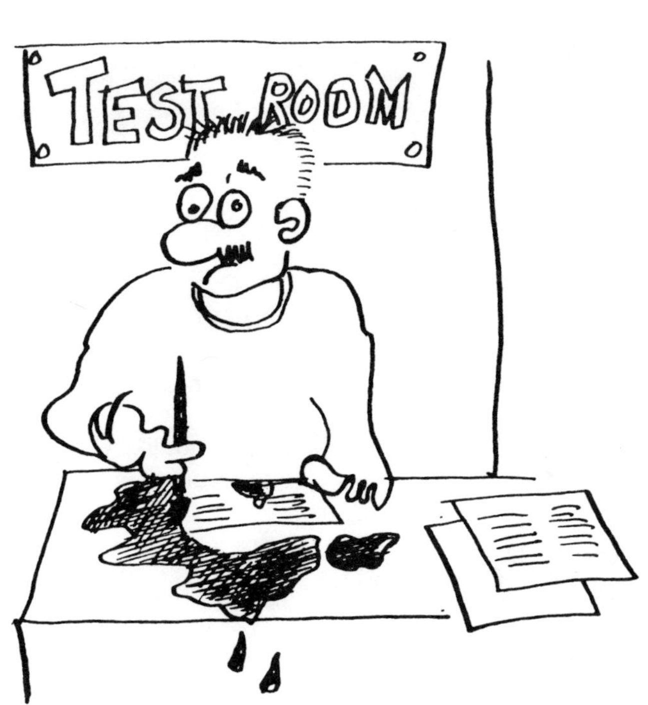

Appendix

a-pen-dix

small sac off
large intestine

A pen that **dix** not work on a **small
stack** will be way off on a **large test**.

C8

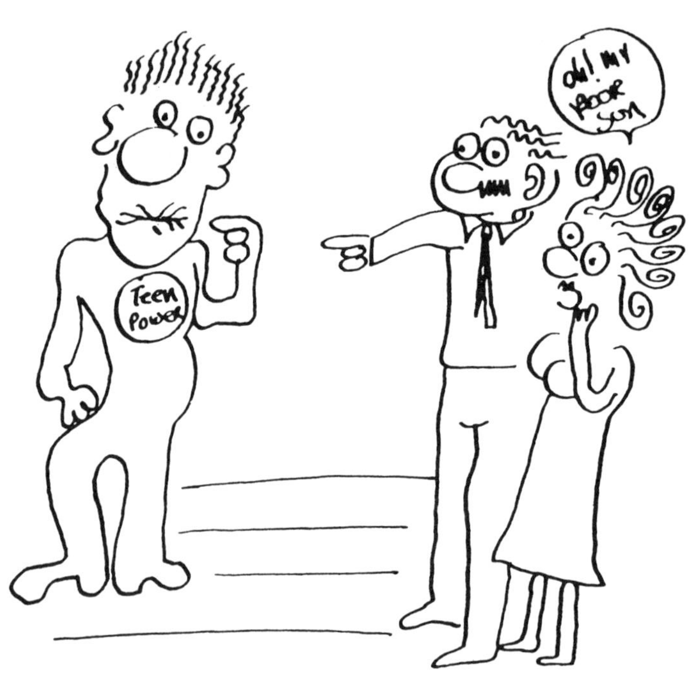

Ascites

a-site-tees

fluid in abdominal
cavity

A sight like **this** teaches us the use
of **fluoride** to prevent **abnormal cavities**.

C9

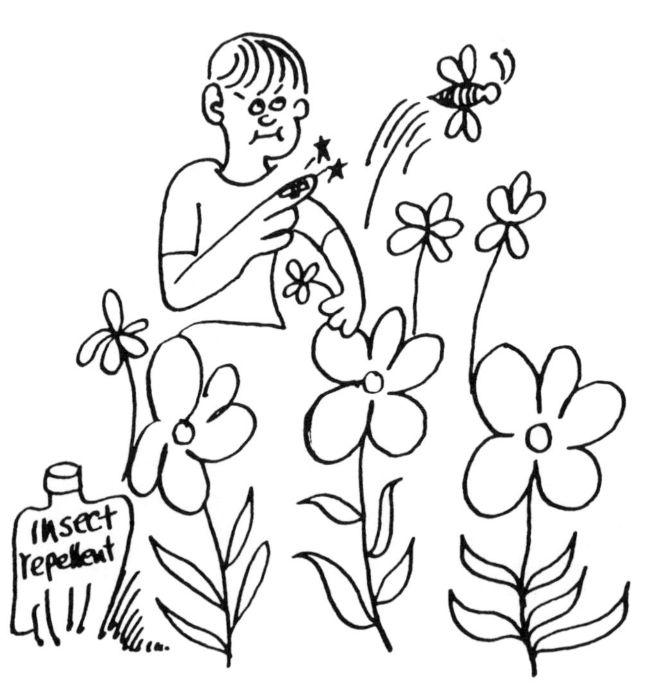

Benign

bee-nine

mild; not likely
to recur

The **bee** bite at **nine** will be
mild and **will not recur**.

C10

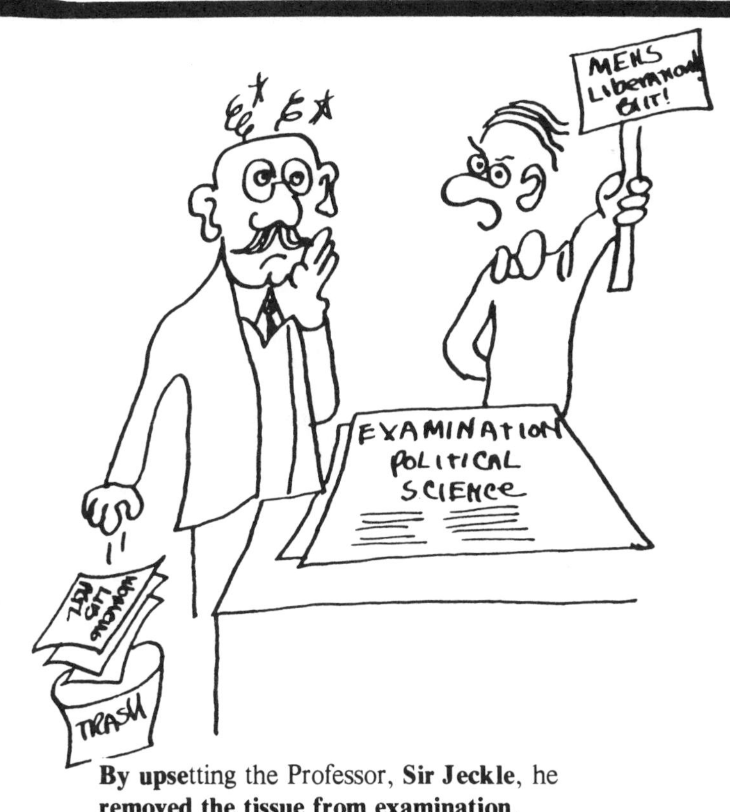

By upsetting the Professor, **Sir Jeckle**, he
removed the tissue from examination.

Biopsy

by-op-see

surgical removal
of tissue for
examination

C11

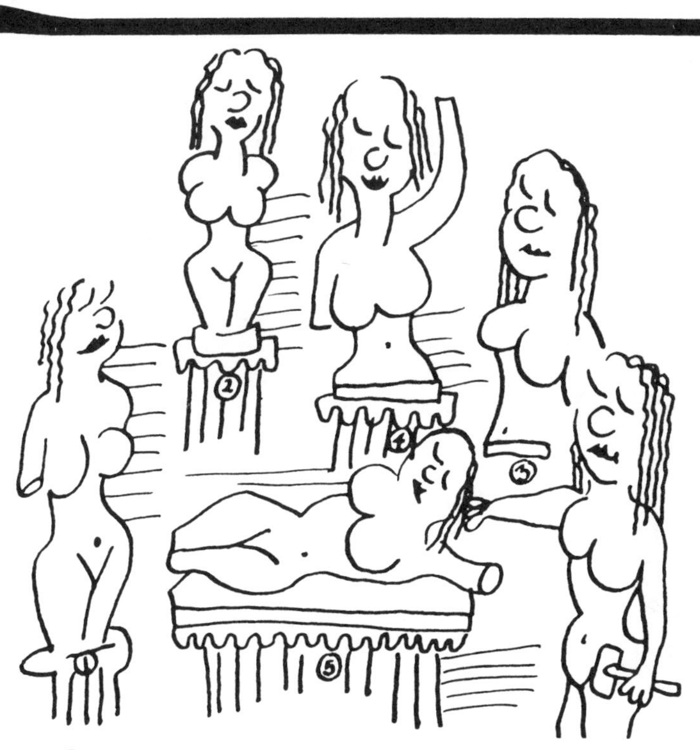

I was **glad her** exact **lik**eness technique
of **sculpturing** was allowed to **domin**ate
the **collection** her works **were in**.

Bladder

blad-der

sac-like structure
in lower abdomen that
collects urine

C12

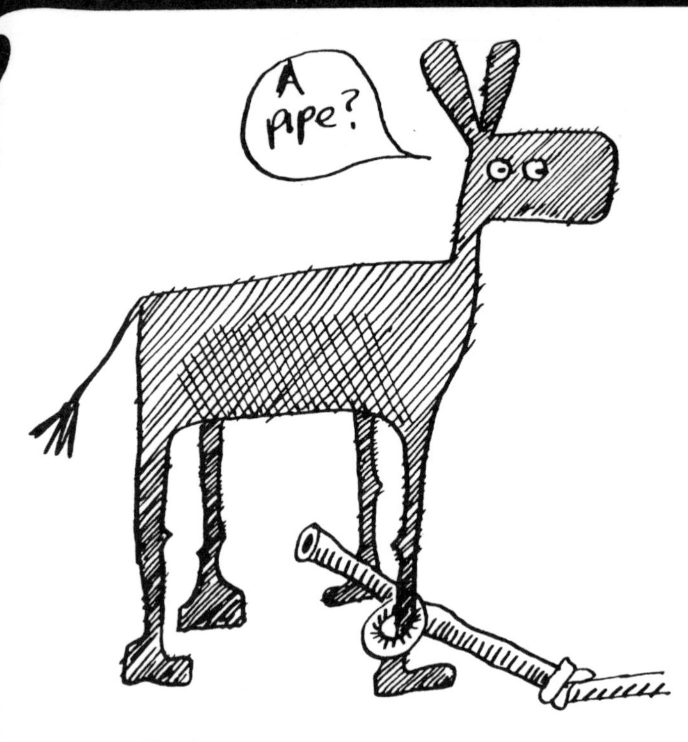

Bronchi

bron-key

windpipes (in lungs)

To tie up a **donkey, wind** a **pipe** around its legs.

C13

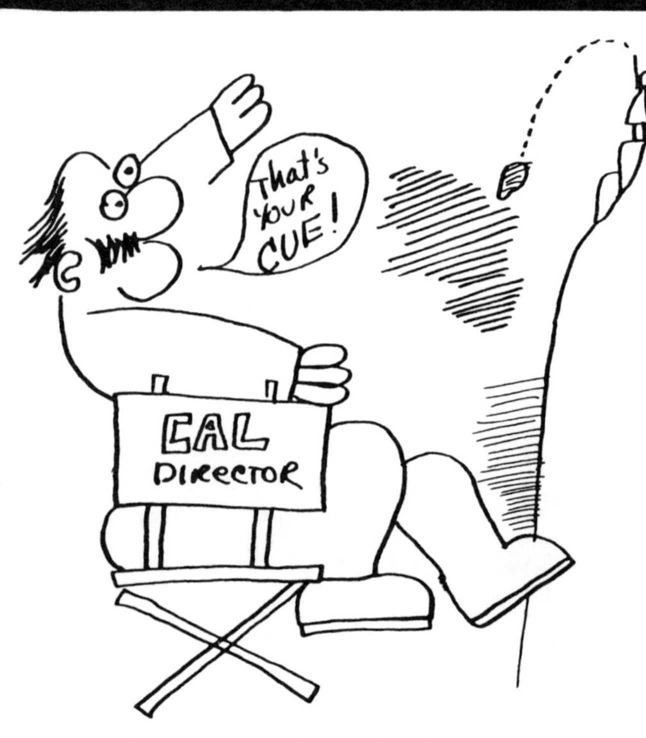

Calculus

cal-cue-lus

stone

The director of the movie, **Cal, cued us** to throw the **stone**.

C14

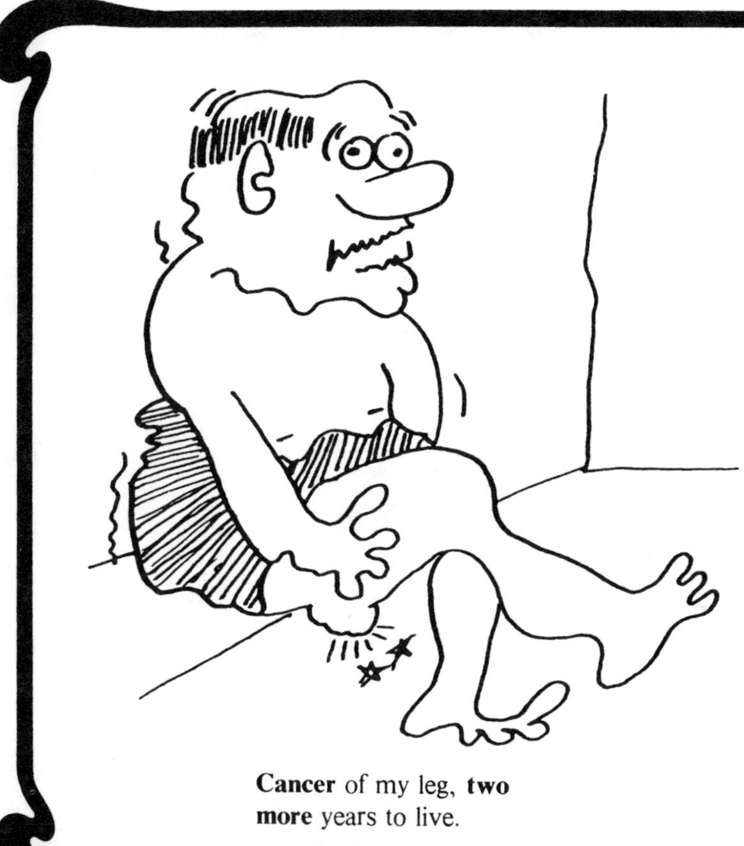

Cancer of my leg, **two more** years to live.

Cancer

kan-sir

malignant tumor

C15

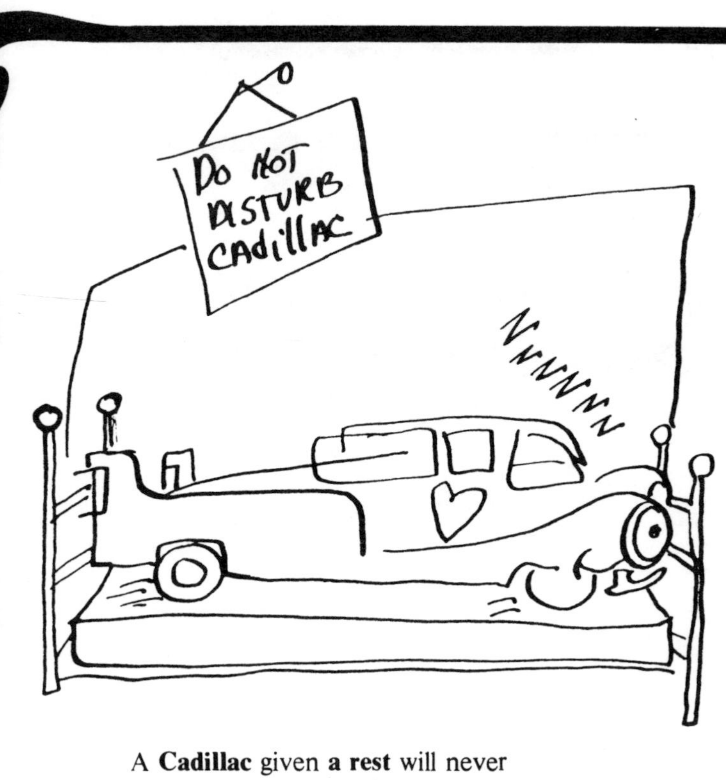

A **Cadillac** given **a rest** will never **stop** running because it has a lot **of heart**.

Cardiac Arrest

kar-dee-ak ah-rest

stoppage of heart

C16

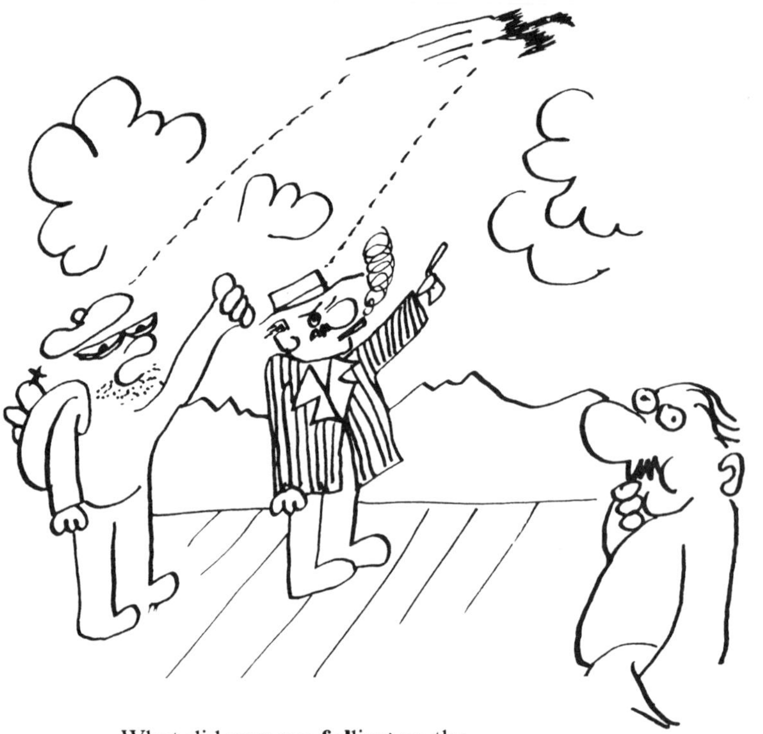

What did you **see fal**ling on the
head of those bad people?

C17

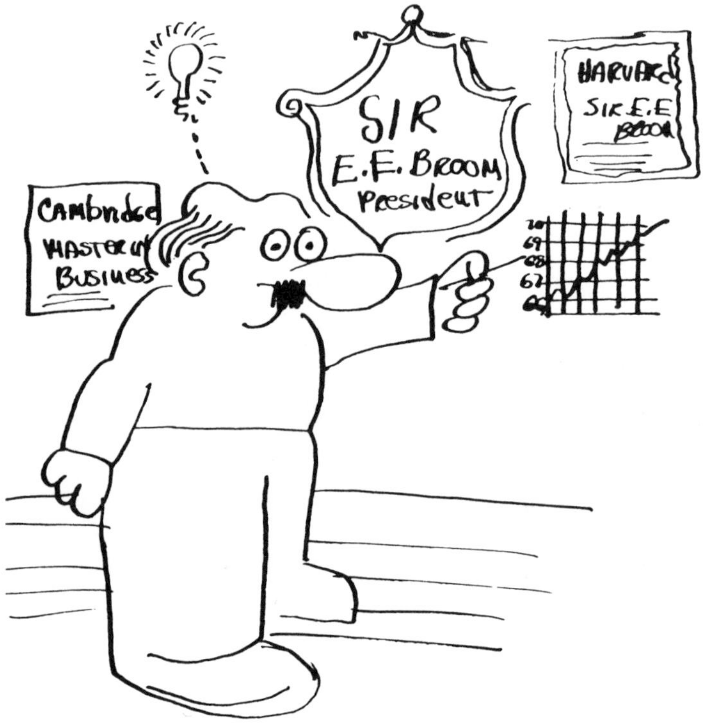

Sir E.E. Broom has a
brilliant **brain** for business.

C18

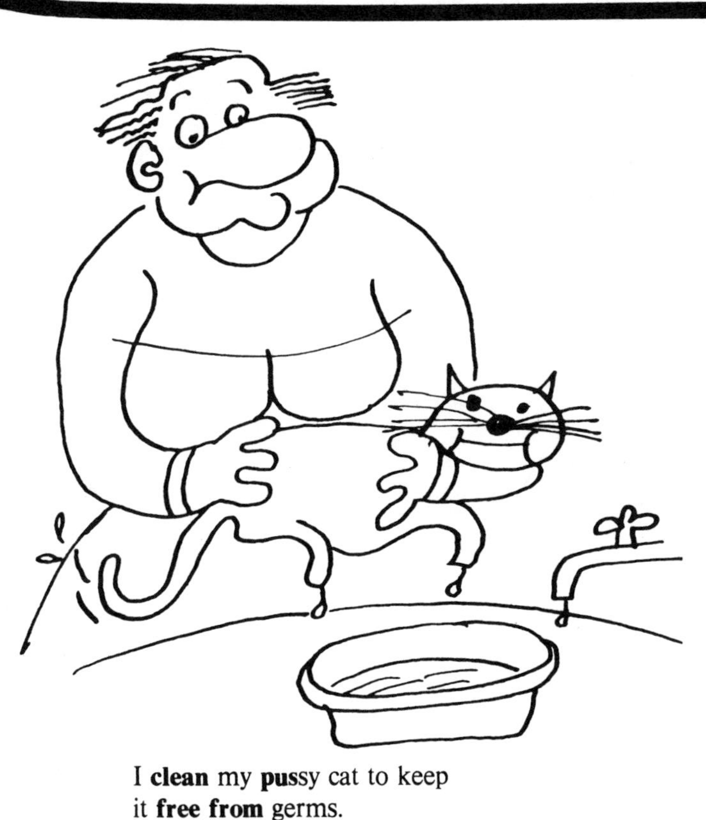

I clean my **pus**sy cat to keep
it **free from** germs.

C19

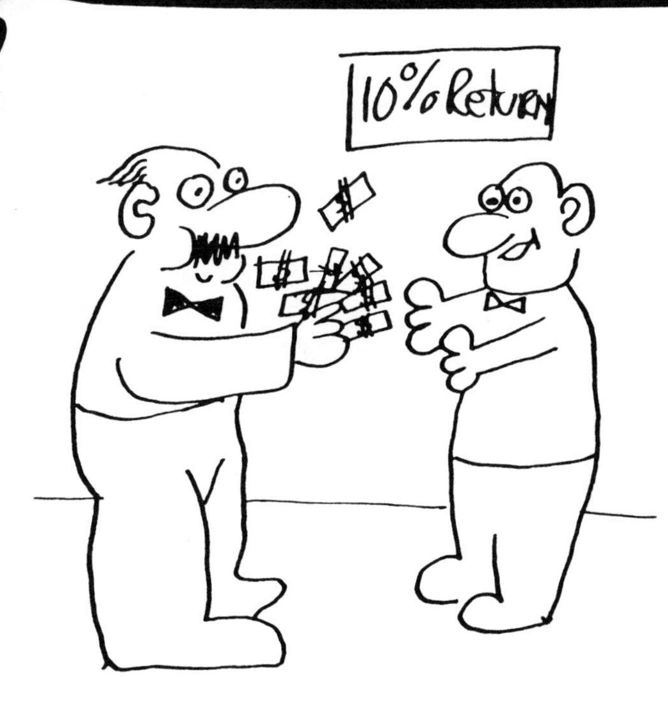

Go lend to companies who pay
large interest in return.

C20

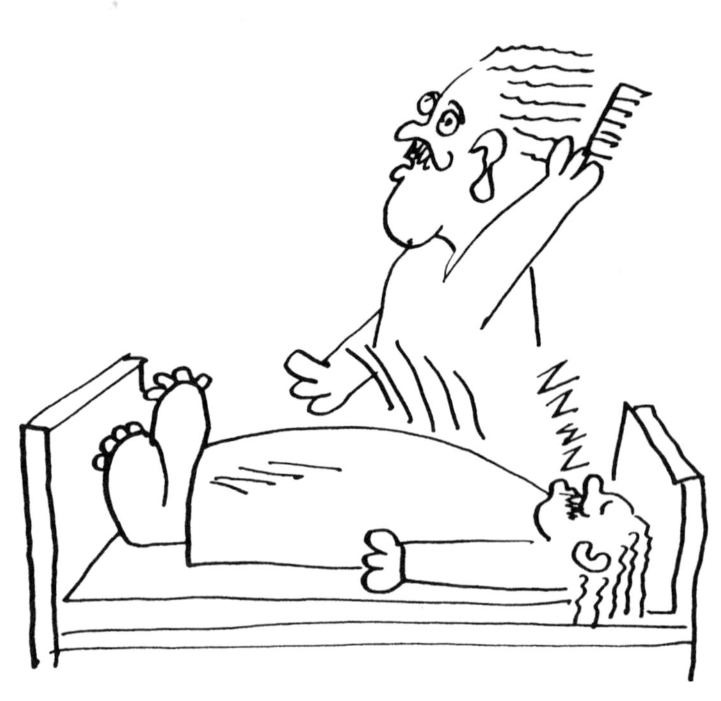

Coma

ko-mah

deep unconsciousness

If I **comb** my hair before I go to
sleep, I will go into **deep
unconsciousness**.

C21

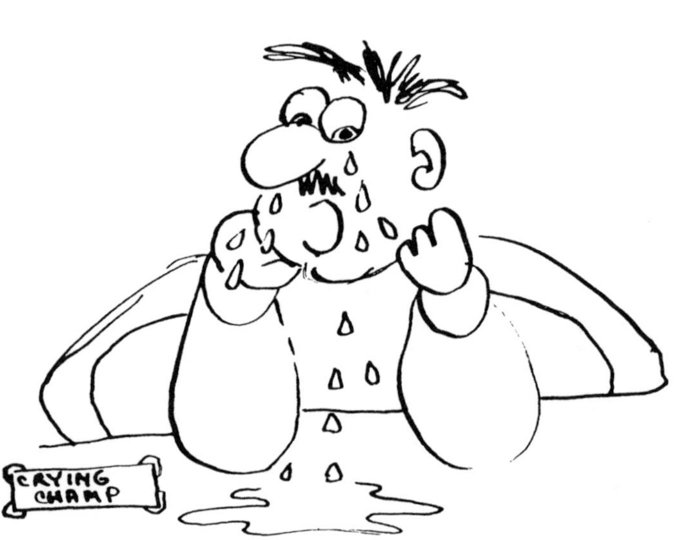

Cranium

cray-nee-um

the skull

His **skill** to **cry**
needs no practice.

C22

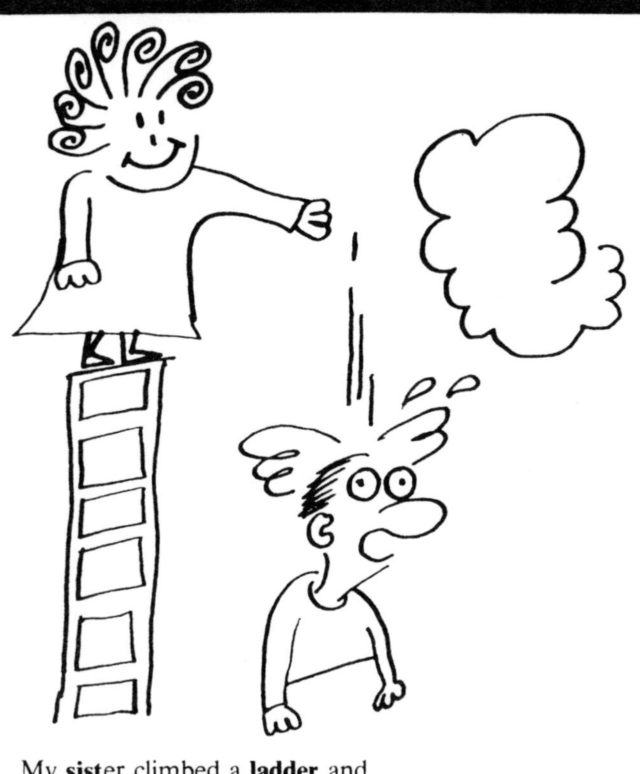

Cyst

sist

bladder-like sac
filled with fluid

My **sist**er climbed a **ladder** and
dropped a **sack with water** on my head.

C23

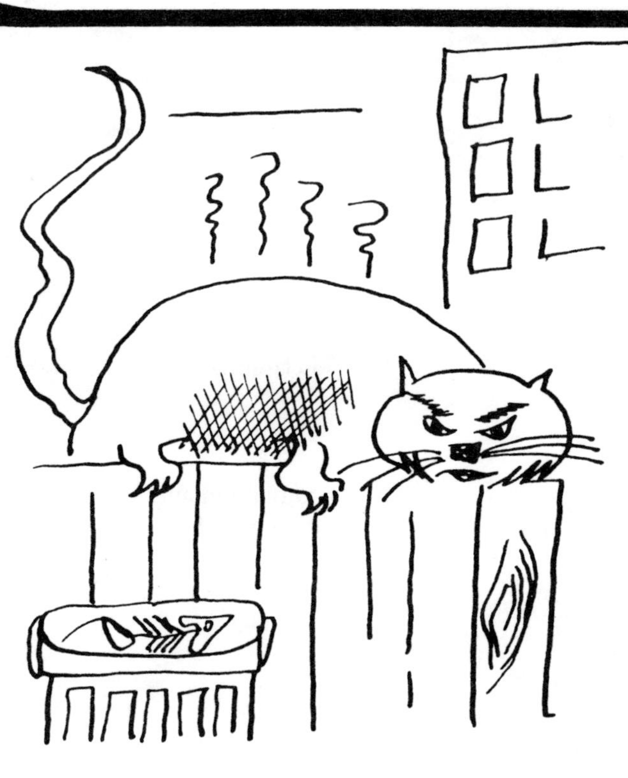

Dirty

dur-tee

containing pus-
producing germs

The **dirty pus**sy cat had **germs** on it.

C24

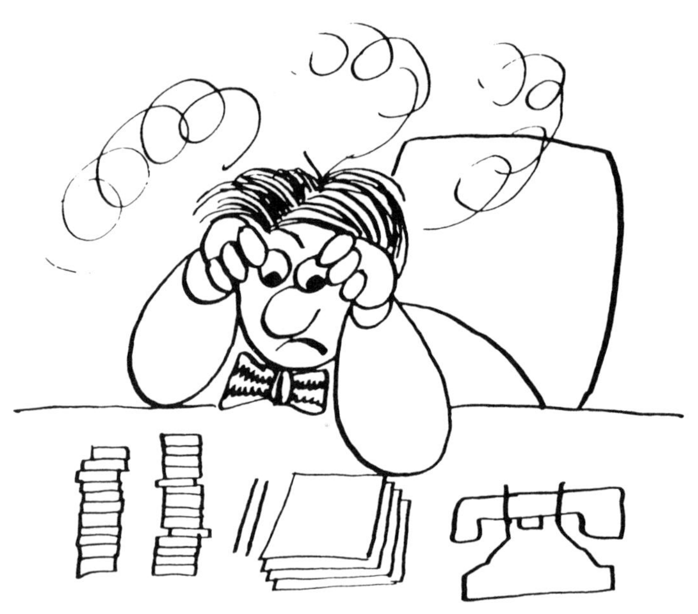

Disease

de-zeeze

sickness

Dis easy job was so dull,
it gave me a **sickness**.

C25

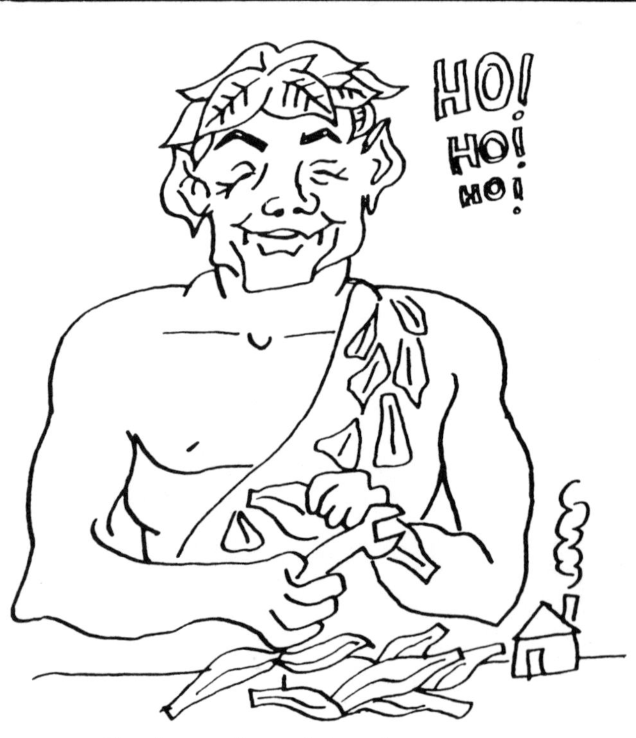

Eclampsia

eh-klamps-e-ah

convulsion after or
before birth

He **clamps the** pods together,
and **convulses** in laughter.

C26

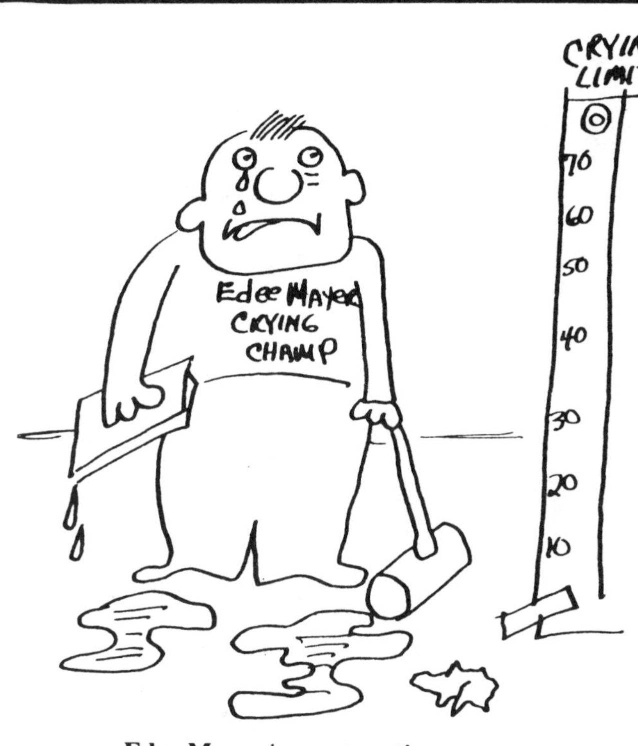

Edema

eh-dee-mah

fluid in tissues

Edee Mayer has watery **tissues**
because he cries a lot.

C27

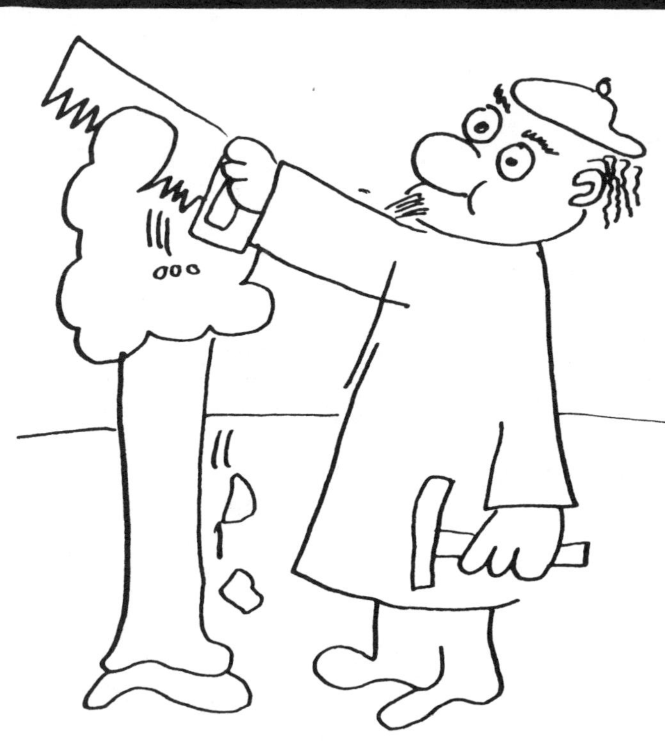

Endoscope

en-doe-skope

instrument used to
look into

In doing sculpture, the **instruments**
he **used looked** like regular tools.

C28

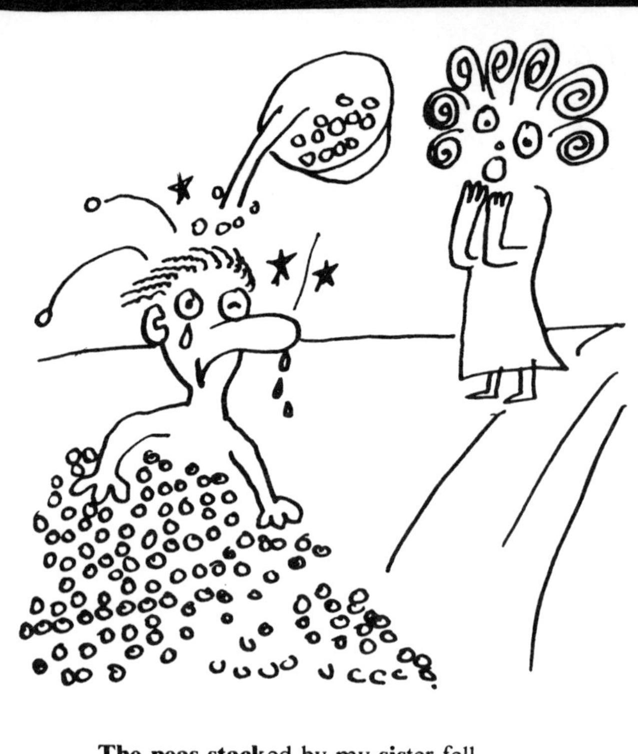

The peas stacked by my **sister** fell
on me and gave me a **nosebleed**.

Epistaxis

eh-pea-stak-siss

nosebleed

C29

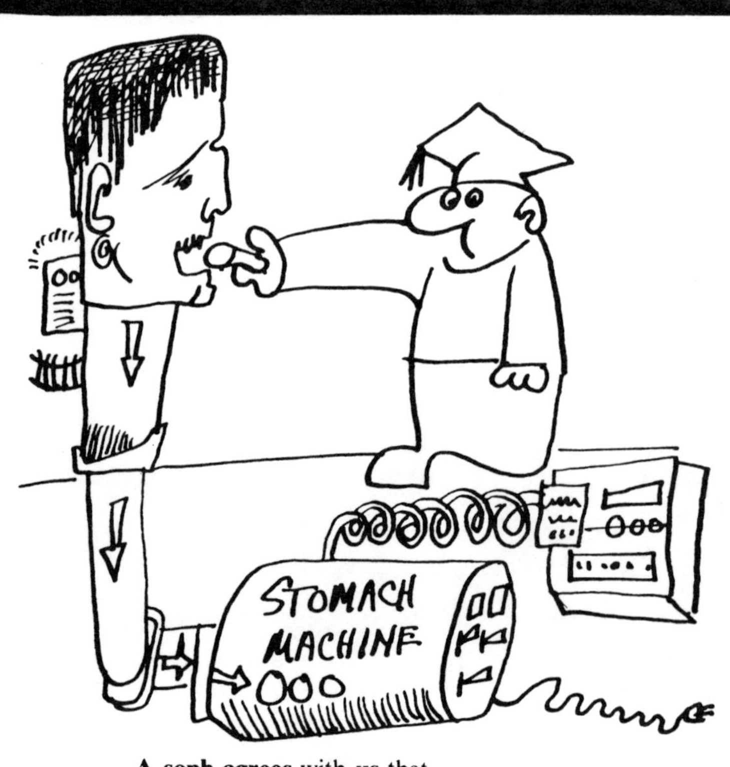

A soph agrees with **us** that
eggs go from **mouth to stomach**.

Esophagus

eh-soph-a-gus

tube connecting
mouth and stomach

C30

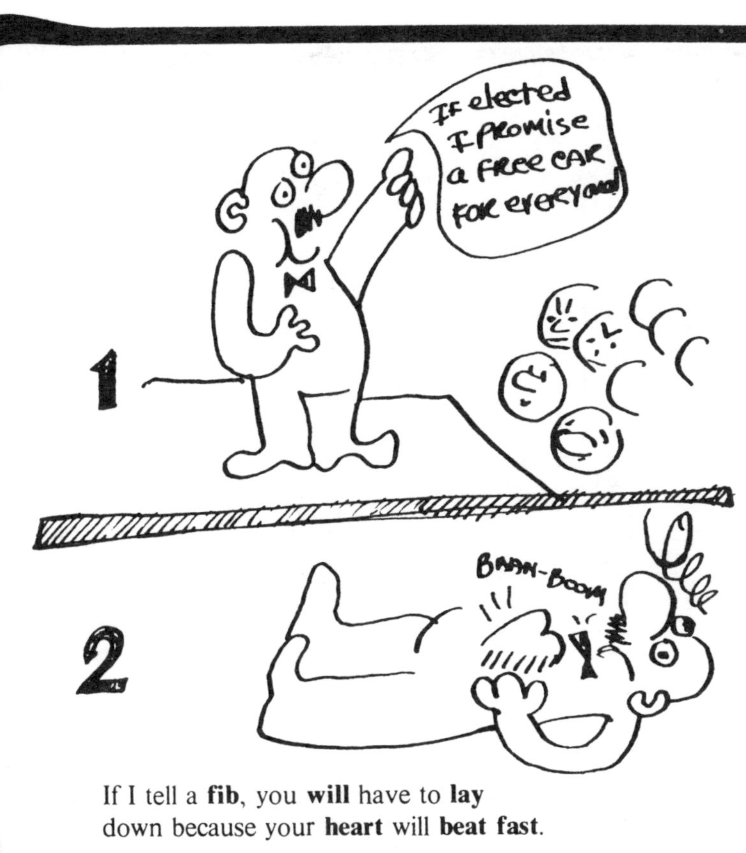

Fibrilla

fib-ril-lay

fast, irregular heartbeat

If I tell a **fib**, you **will** have to **lay** down because your **heart** will **beat fast**.

C31

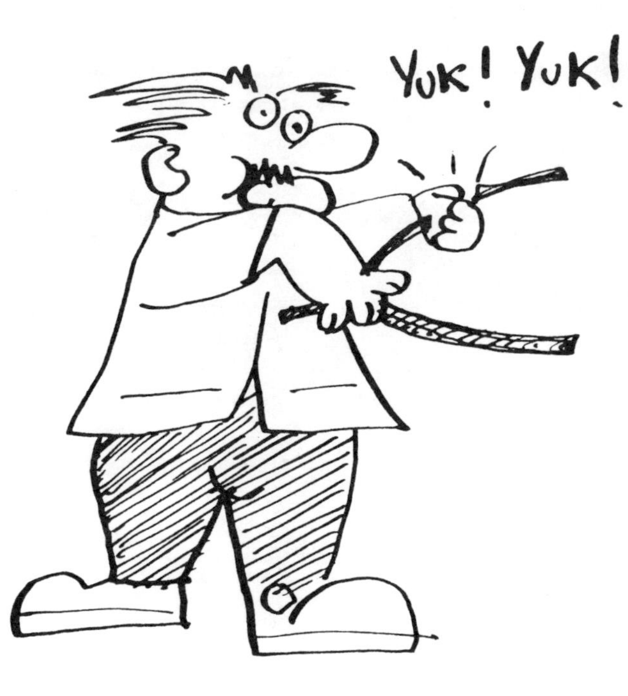

Fracture

frack-shure

crack or break in bone

Mr. **Frack sure** made a funny **crack** about the wish**bone**.

C32

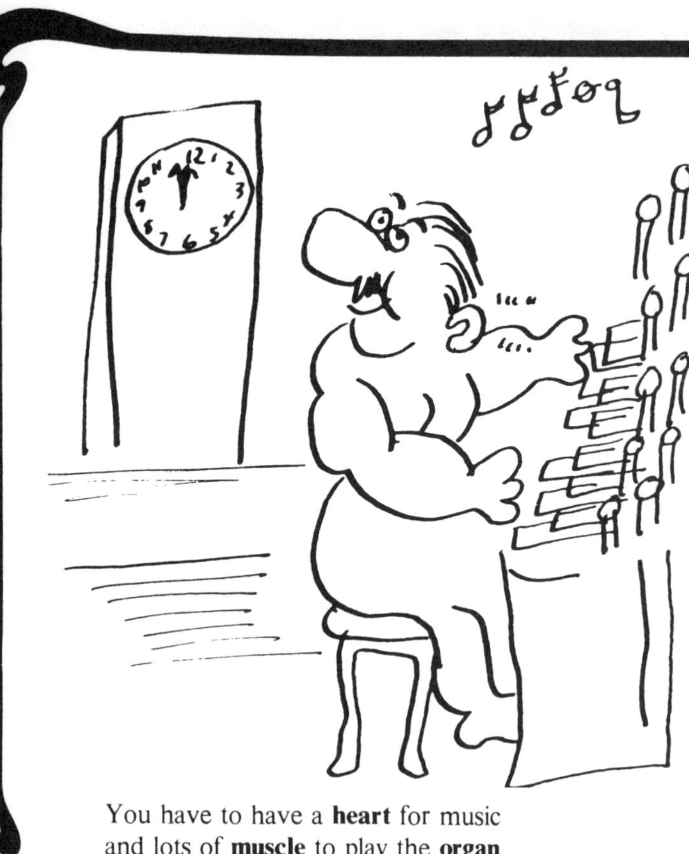

Heart

hart

muscular organ
between lungs

You have to have a **heart** for music
and lots of **muscle** to play the **organ**.

C33

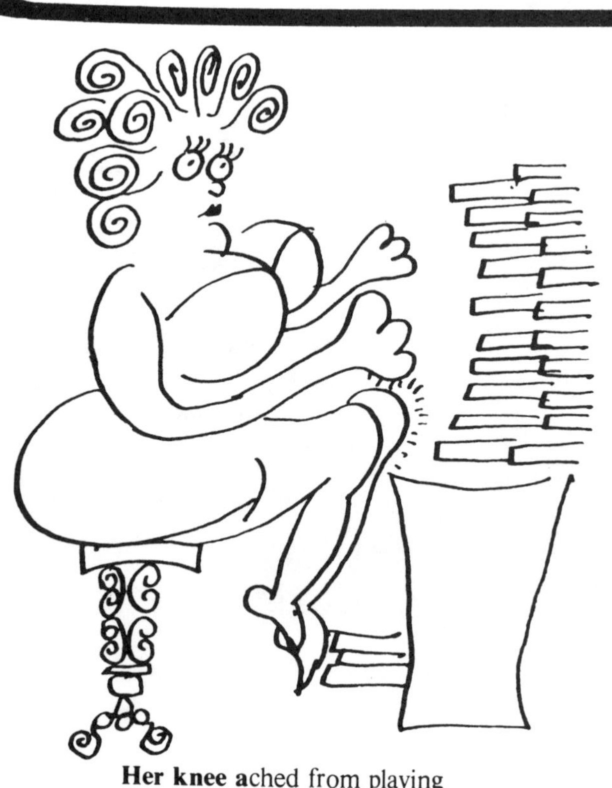

Hernia

her-nee-ah

protrusion of organ
through lining

Her knee ached from playing
a **profusion of organ** pieces.

C34

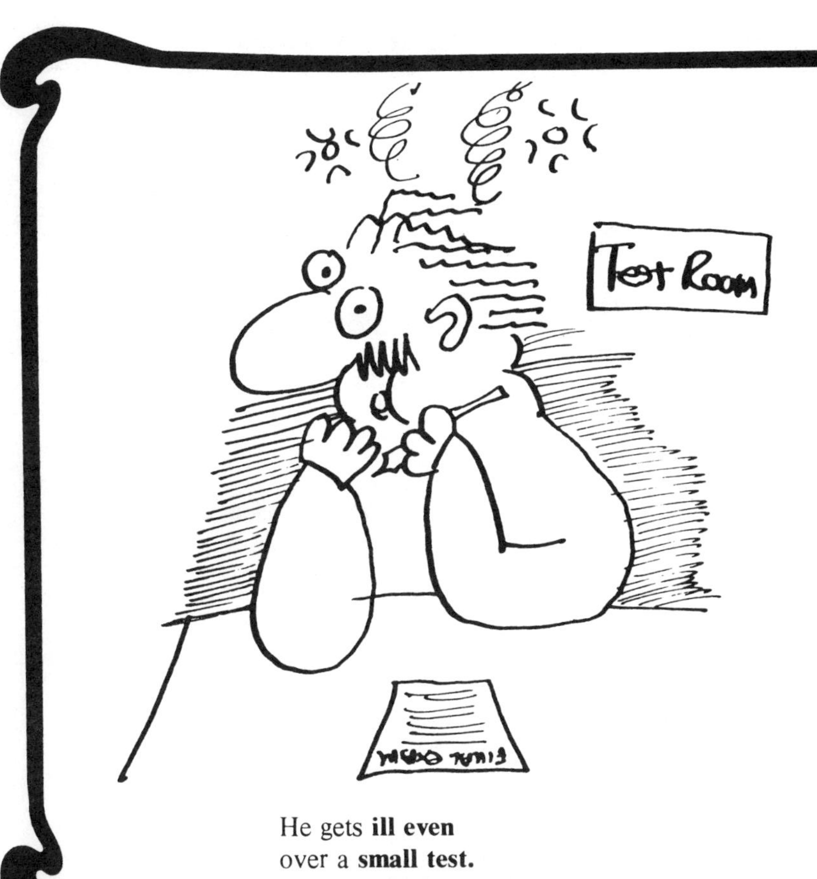

He gets **ill even** over a **small test.**

C35

Ileum

ill-ee-um

small intestine

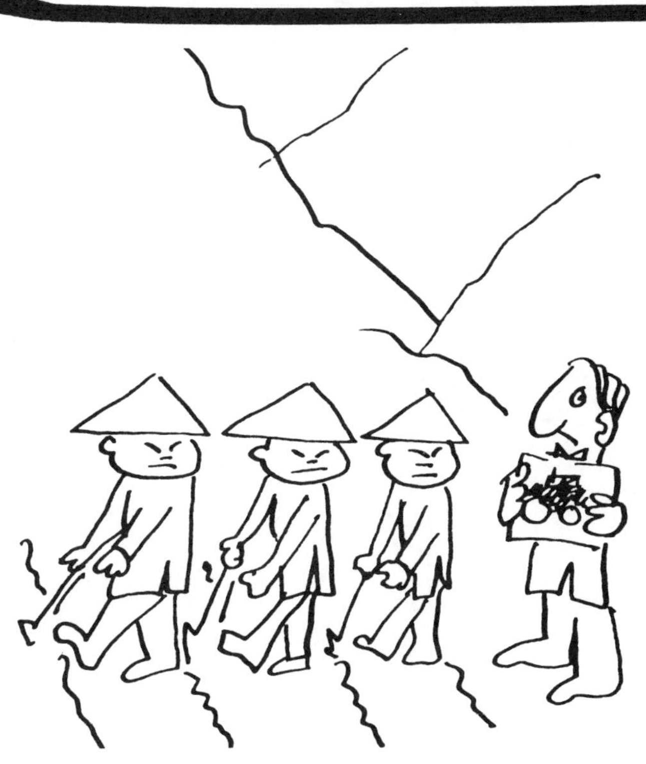

In a **test in** the **low** lands, Reader's **Digest** found **tract**ors were not popular.

C36

Intestine

in-tess-tin

lower digestive tract

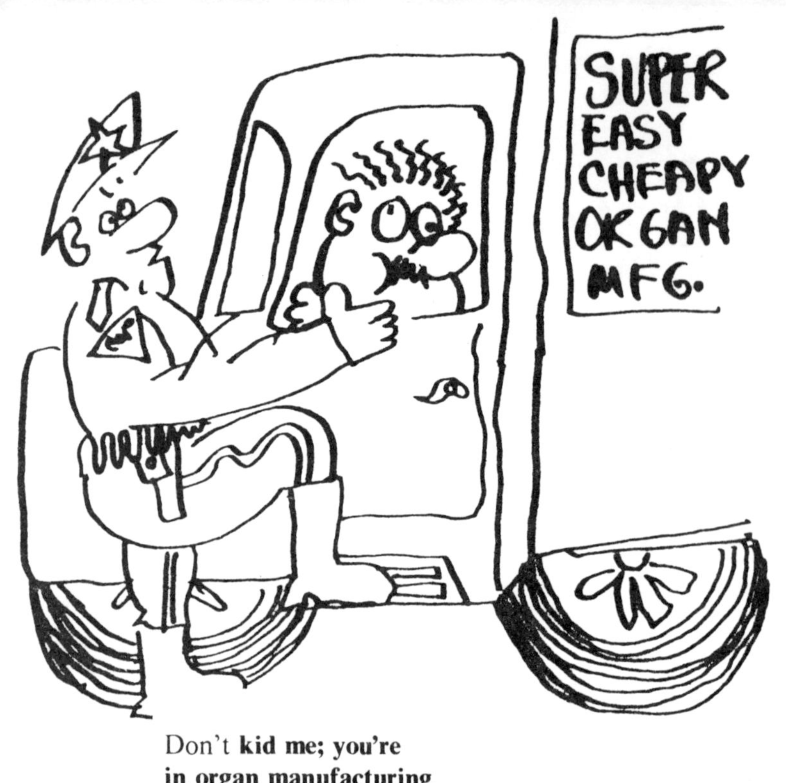

Kidney

kid-nee

organ that manufactures
urine

Don't **kid me; you're
in organ manufacturing**.

C37

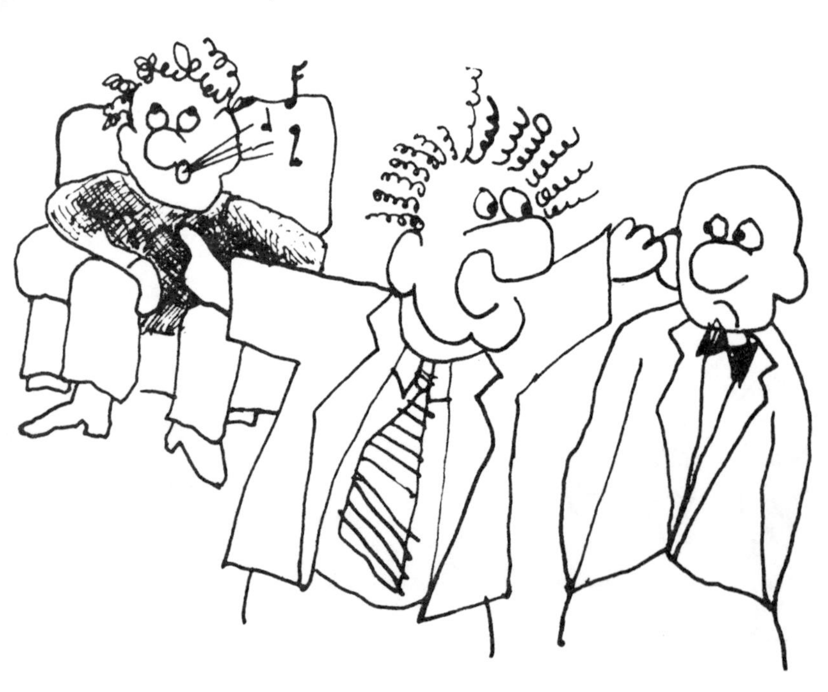

Lesion

lee-shun

diseased tissue

Lee, shun dat man who won't
agree dat **dis is de issue**.

C38

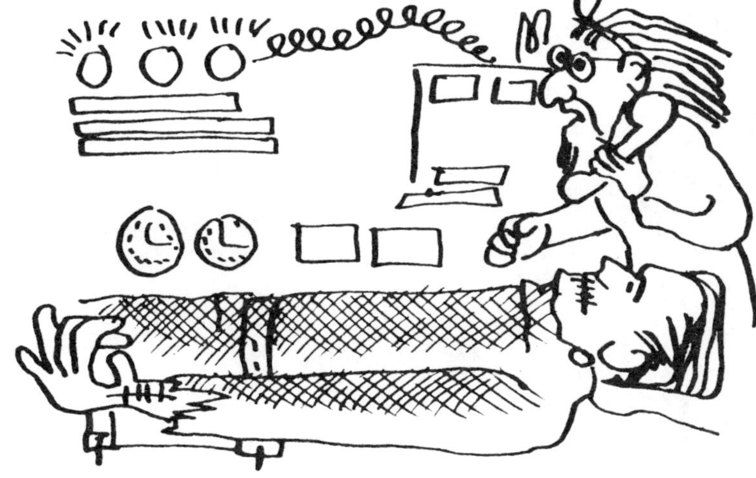

Deliver the parts and I will **manufacture** an **organ** in the mean**while.**

C39

Liver

live-er

organ that manufactures bile

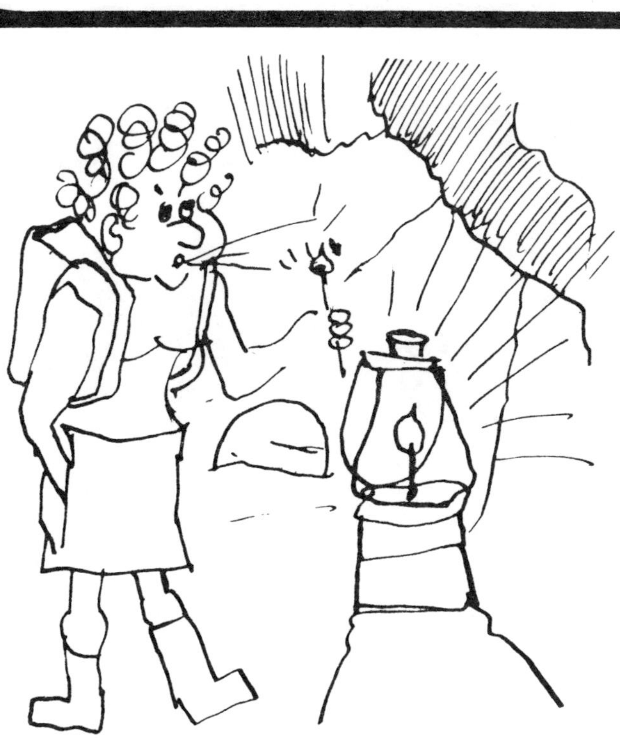

She **lit the a**rc lamp so that she could see the strange **stone formations.**

C40

Lithia

lith-ee-ah

formation of stone

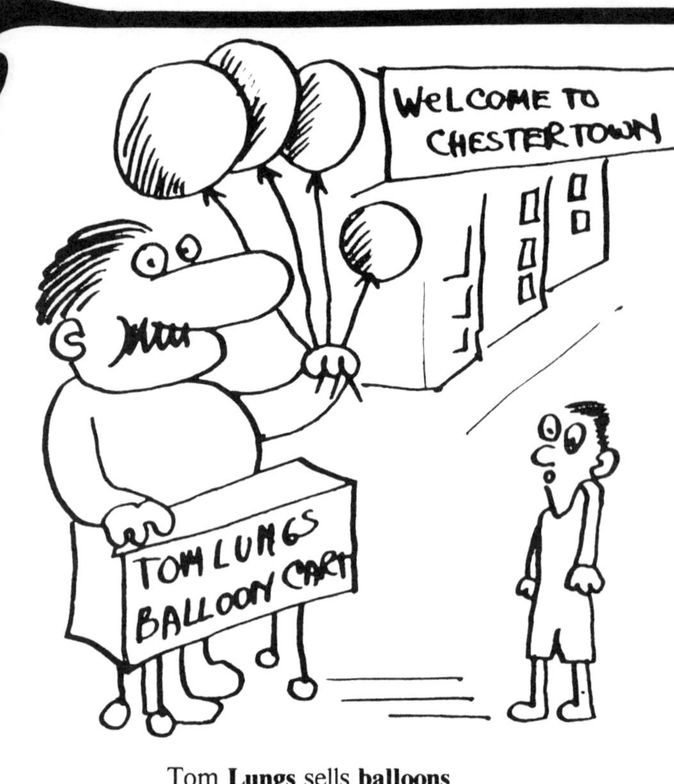

Tom **Lungs** sells **balloons**
in **Chest**ertown, Pa.

Lungs

lungs

balloon-like organs
in the chest

C41

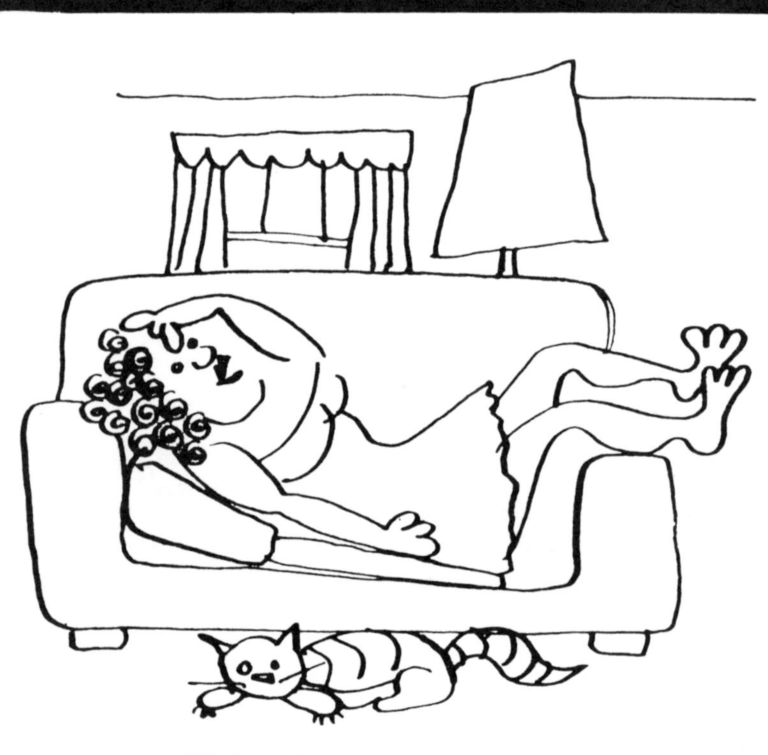

Ma lays down when she
does **not feel well**.

Malaise

mal-aze

not well; a feeling
of illness

C42

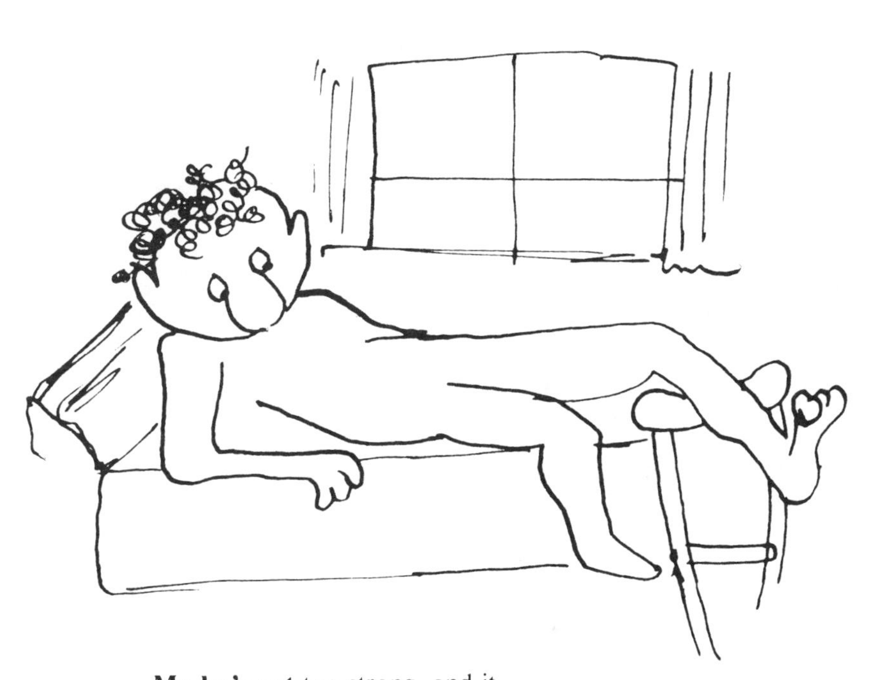

Malignant

mah-lig-nant

tending to grow worse
and to recur

My leg's not too strong, and it
seems **to grow worse** every year.

C43

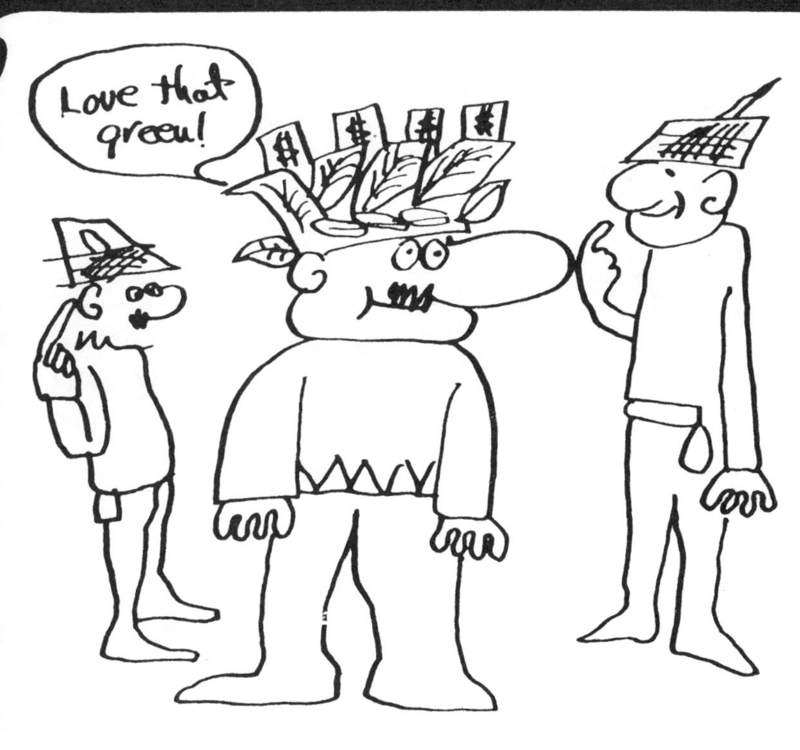

Meninges

men-in-gees

brain covering

Men enjoy green hats
that **cover** their **brains**.

C44

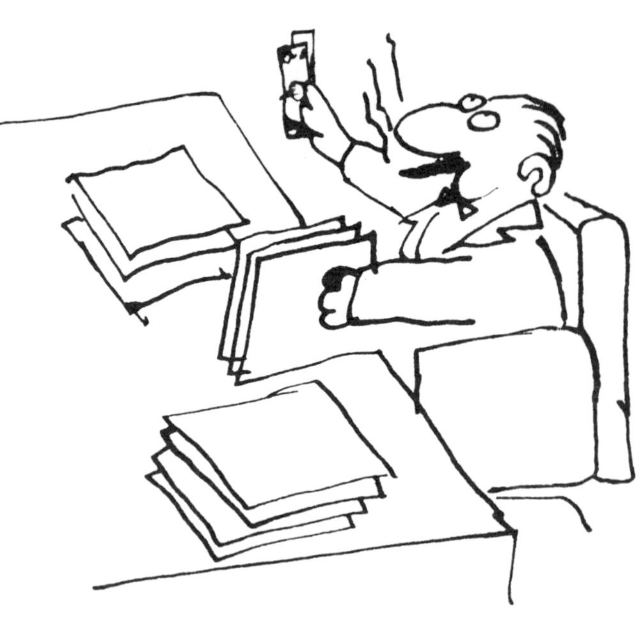

Neoplasm

knee-o-plaz-em

growth of tissue
with no purpose

There is **no purpose** to the **growing issu**ance
of bills, but **Neal pays 'em** anyway.

C45

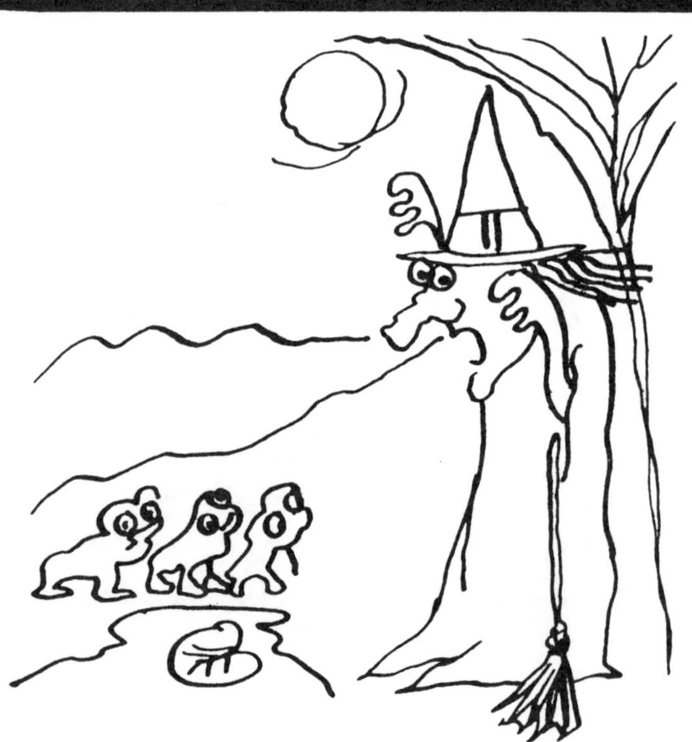

Ovary

oh-va-ree

sex gland producing
human egg

Over each a hex was **plan**ned to
make them **produce human eggs**.

C46

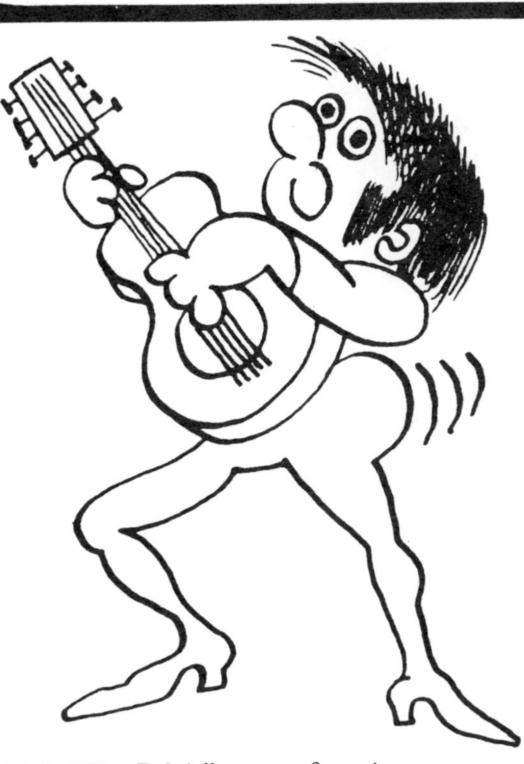

Pelvis

pel-vis

basin-shaped bones
of lower trunk

Elvis ''The **Pelvis''** rose to fame by
shaking the **bones in** his **lower trunk**.

C47

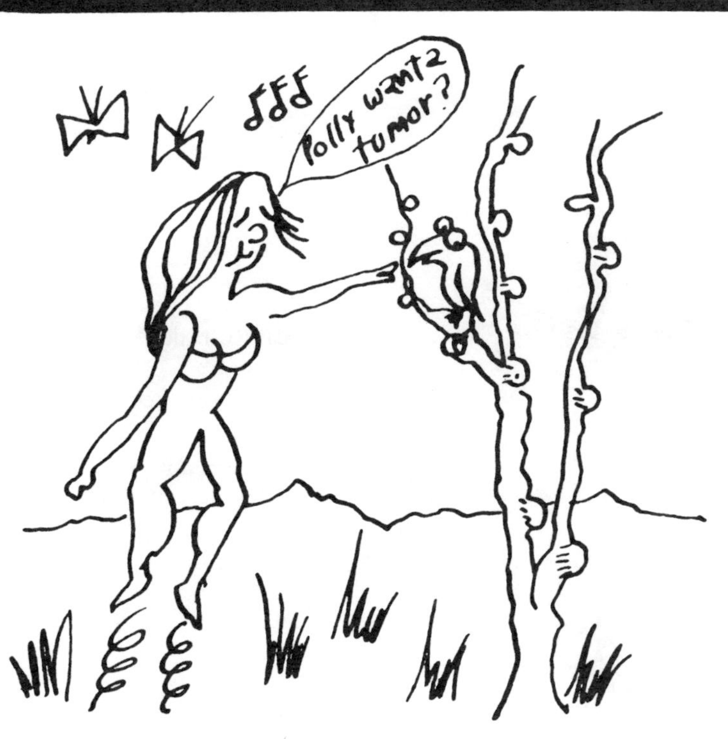

Polyp

pol-lip

tumor on a stem

Polly the **Imp** picked
tumors off the **stems**.

C48

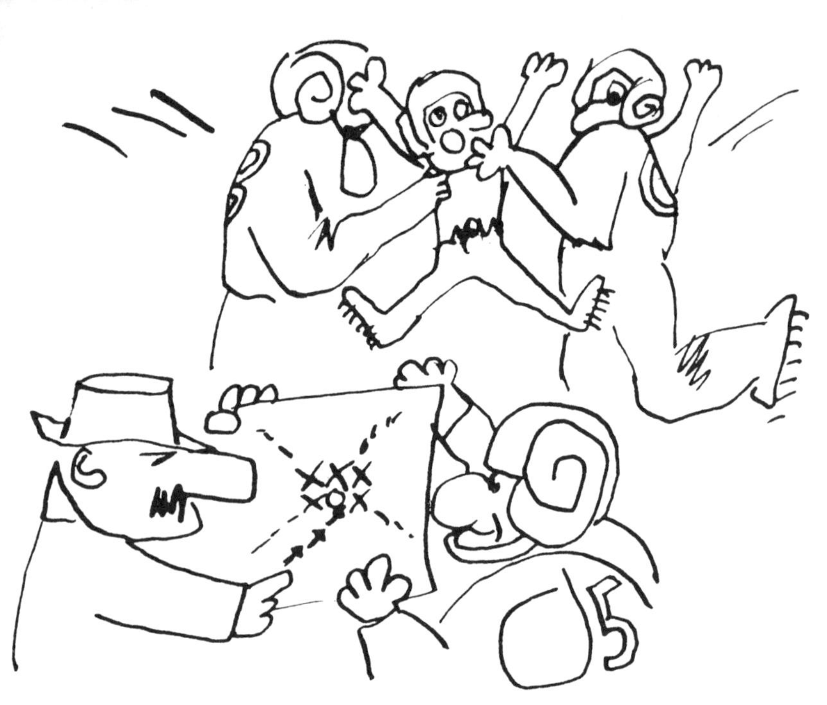

Prostate

pross-tate

gland surrounding neck
of the bladder

The **pros state** in their game **plans** that they
intend to **surround the necks of the "blad"** guys.

C49

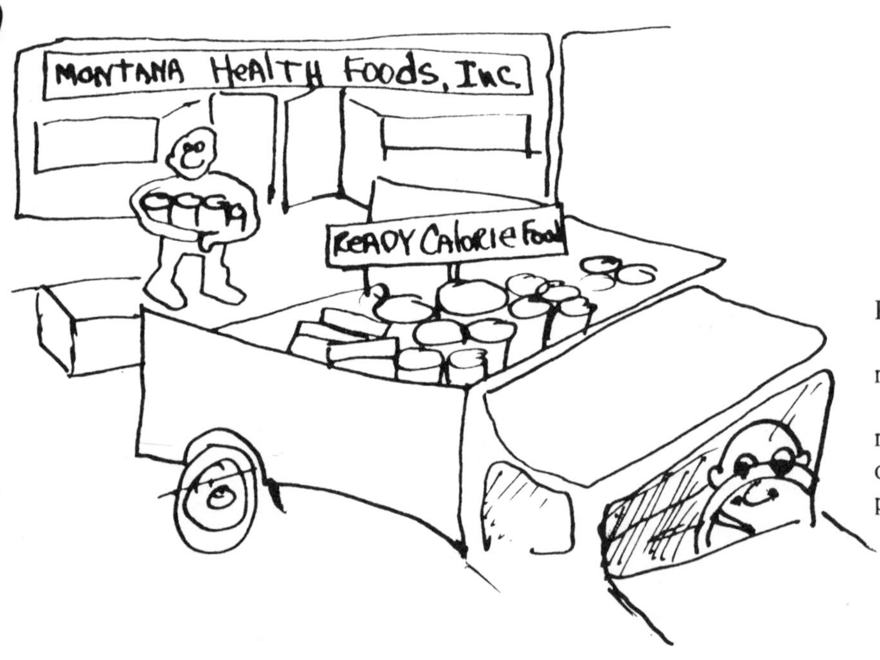

Radical Resection

rad-ee-kal ree-seck-shun

removal by surgery of
organ and surrounding
parts

The **ready-calorie section** of Montana Health
Foods was **removed** (because it was too **sugary**)
to **Oregon**.

C50

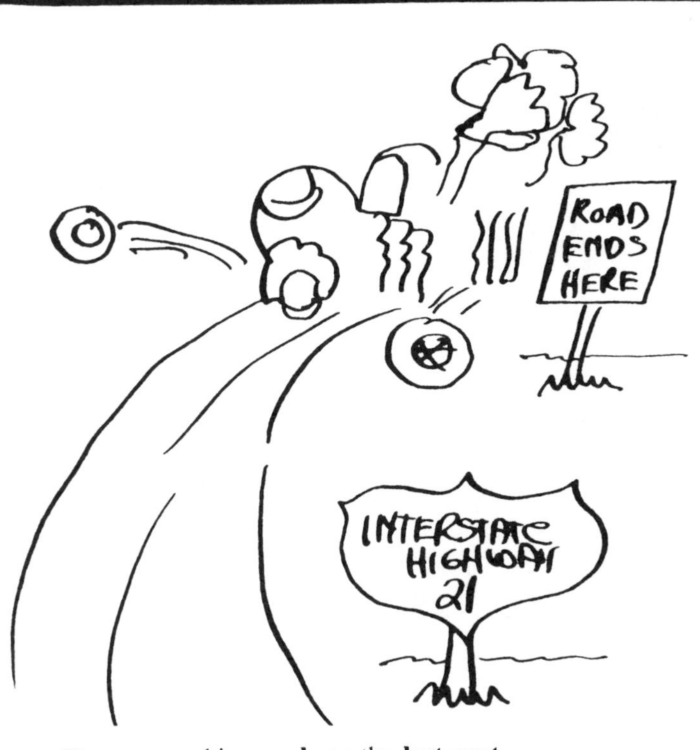

There was a big **wreck on** the **last part** of the **large interstate** highway.

Rectum

reck-tum

last part of large intestine

C51

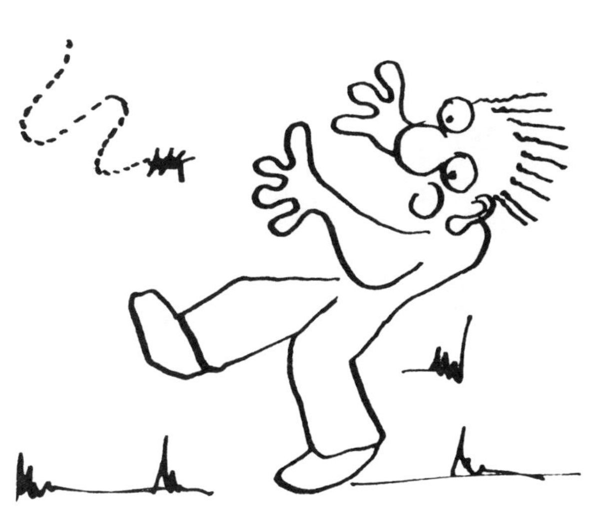

A **sick tick** has **pus-producing germs**.

Septic

sep-tick

pus-producing germs

C52

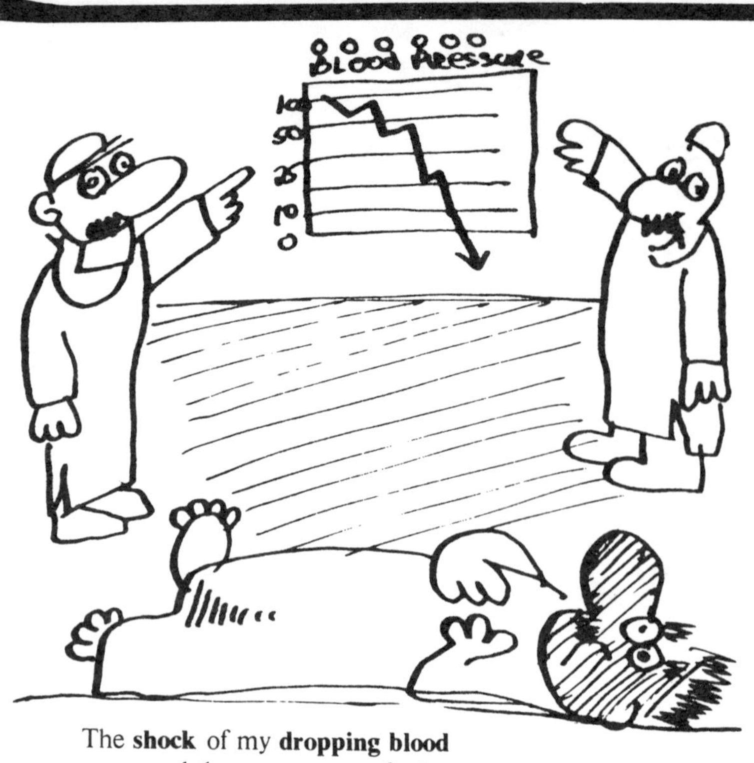

Shock

shock

drop in blood pressure
after injury or
operation

The **shock** of my **dropping blood
pressure**d them to prevent further
injury after the operation.

C53

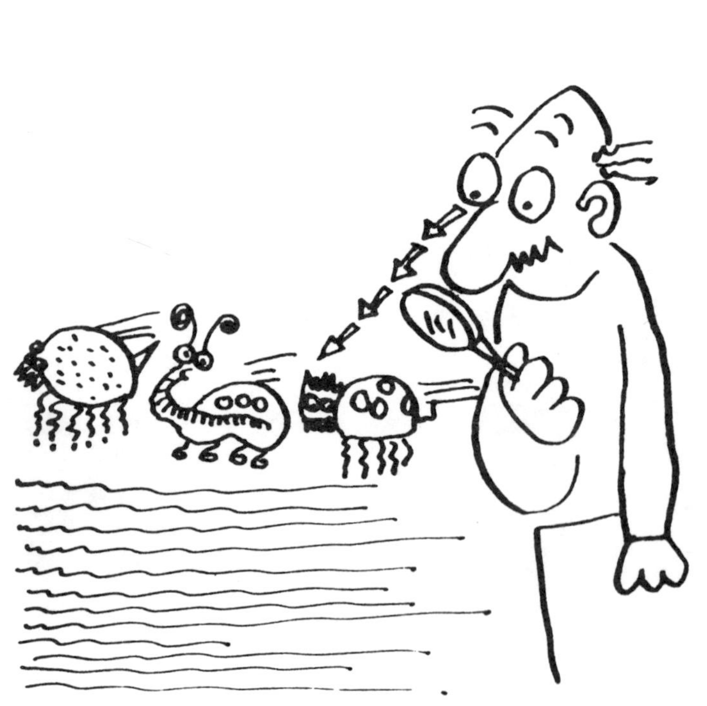

Sterile

stair-ul

free of all living
germs

Stare at **ill** bugs and they go
away, leaving you **free of germs**.

C54

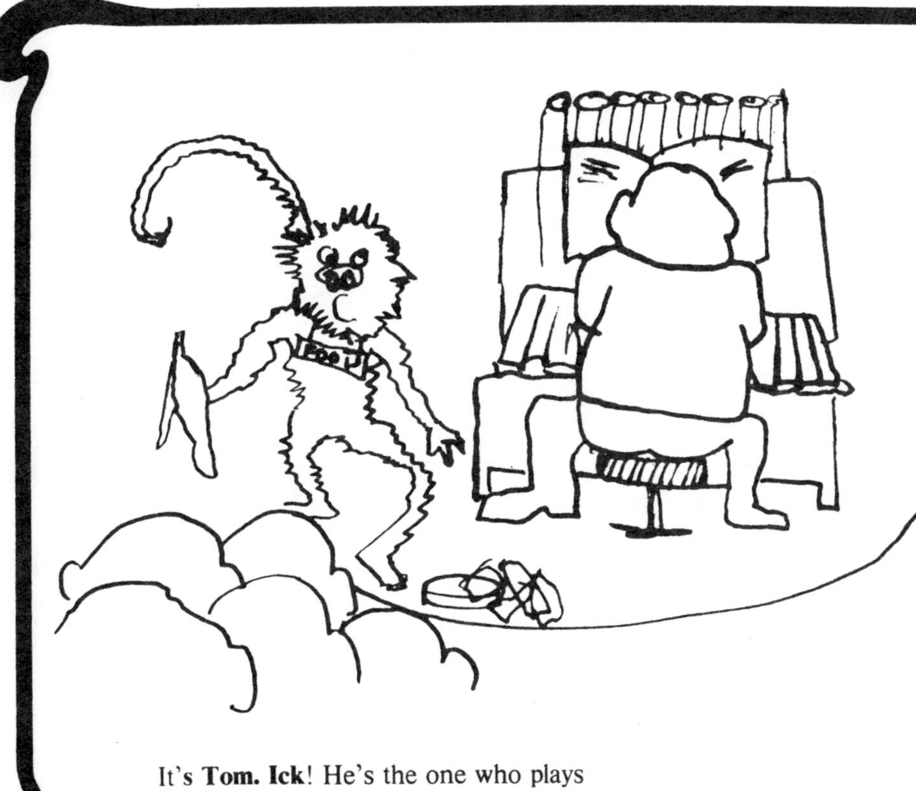

Stomach

stum-ik

elastic organ that
collects food

It's **Tom. Ick**! He's the one who plays
the **organ** while his monkey **collects food**.

C55

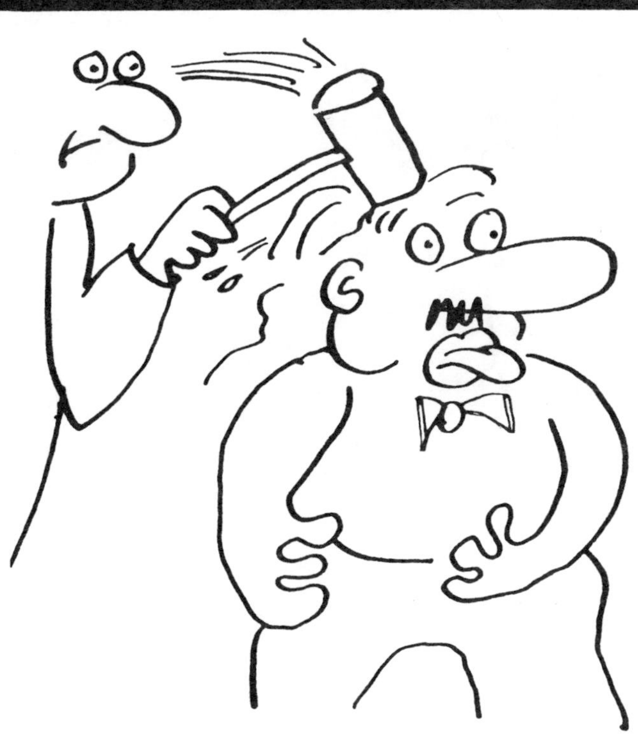

Stroke

stroke

bursting of blood
vessel in brain

A **stroke** on the head and
the **blood vessel broke**.

C56

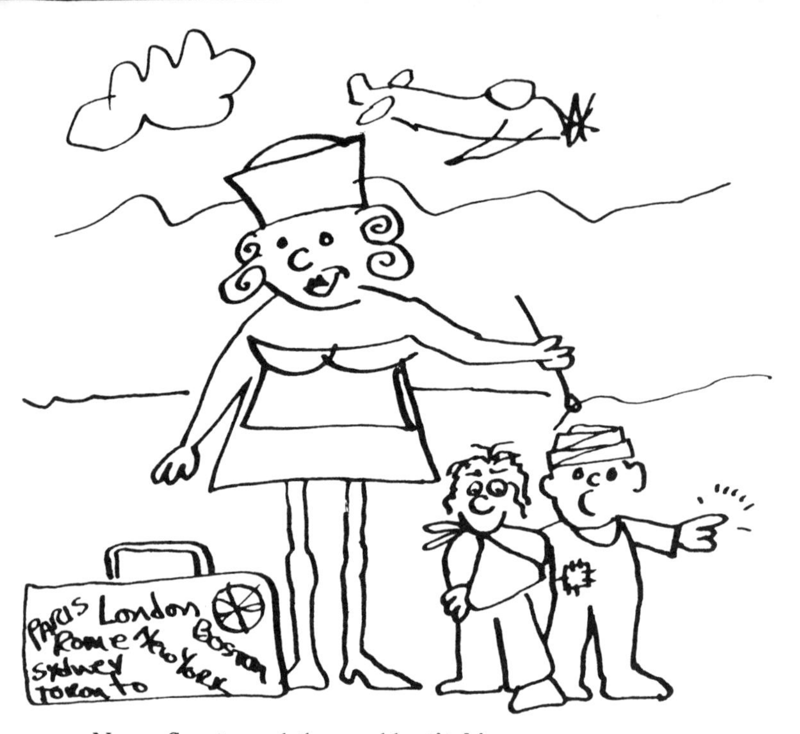

Suture

sue-tour

stitch to close a wound

Nurse **Sue tour**ed the world, **stitching clothes** and healing **wounds**.

C57

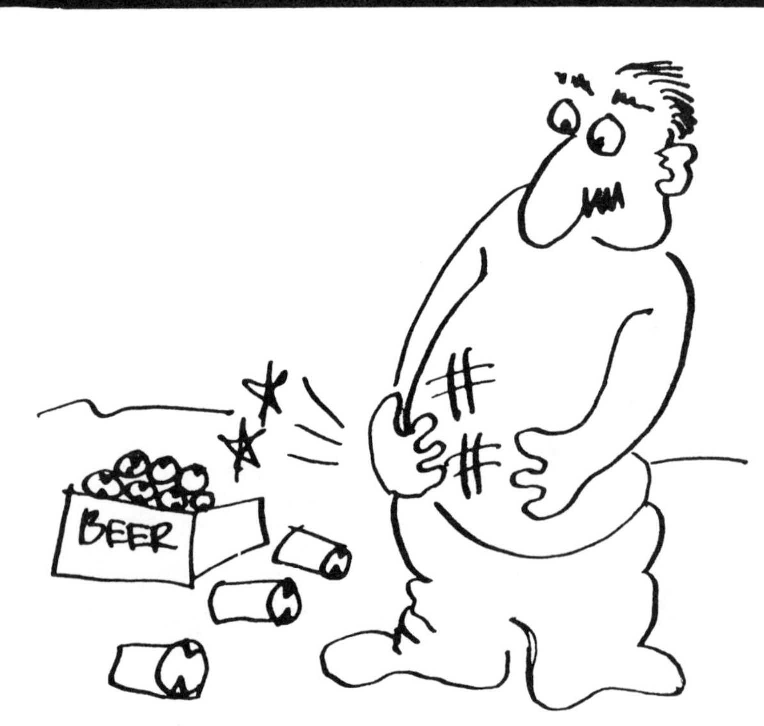

Symptom

simp-tum

sign of disease

A **simple tum**my ache
can be a **sign of disease.**

C58

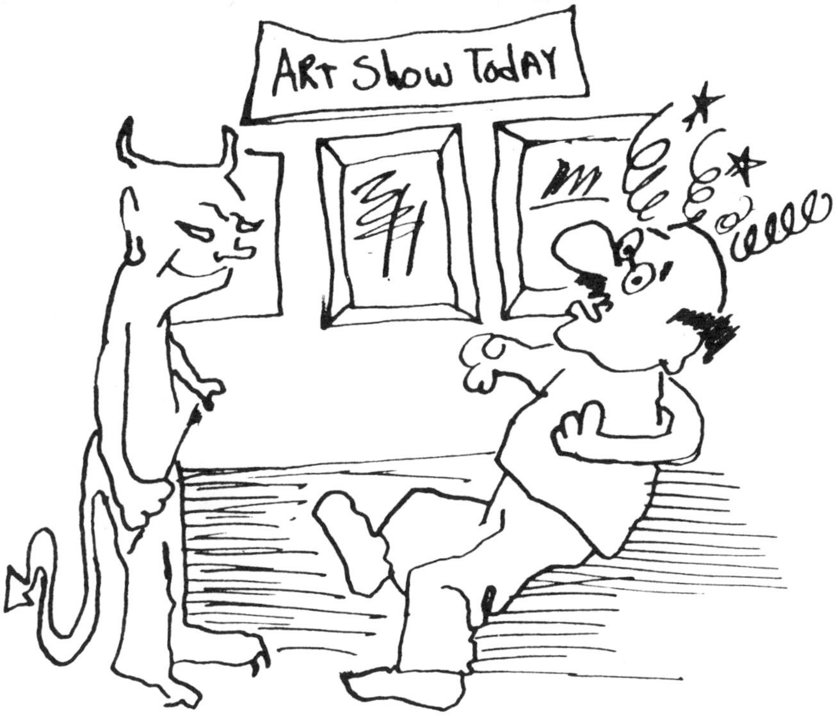

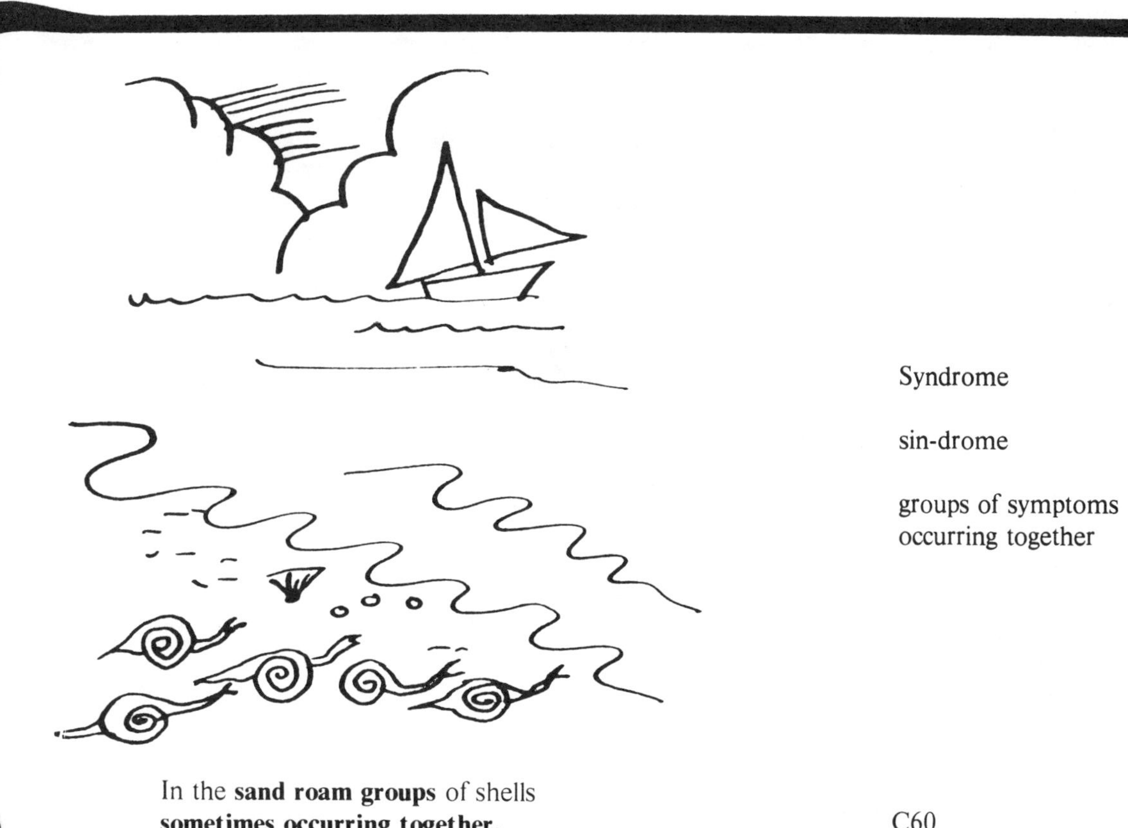

Syncope

sin-cope

fainting

It's a **sin** to **cope** with the
painting being done today.

C59

Syndrome

sin-drome

groups of symptoms
occurring together

In the **sand roam groups** of shells
sometimes occurring together.

C60

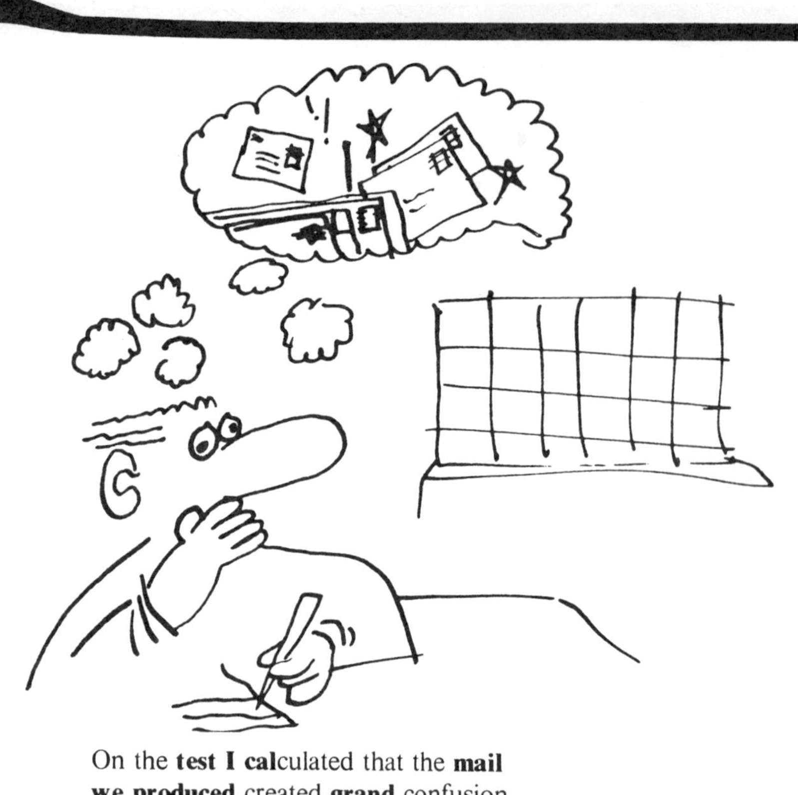

Testicle

tess-ti-kal

male reproductive
sex gland

On the **test I calc**ulated that the **mail
we produced** created **grand** confusion
last year.

C61

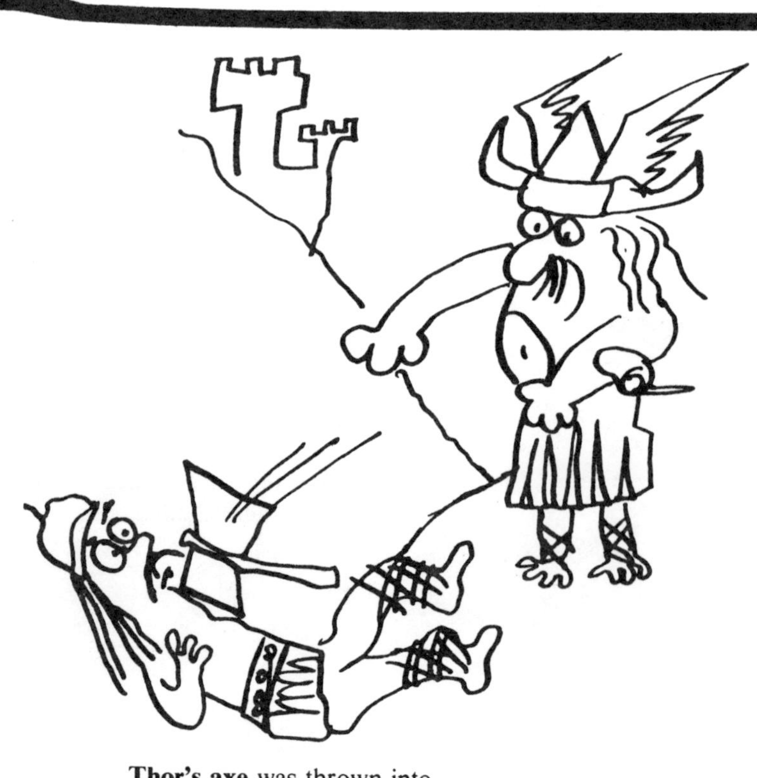

Thorax

thor-axe

bony cage of the chest

Thor's axe was thrown into
the **cage of the** villain's **chest**.

C62

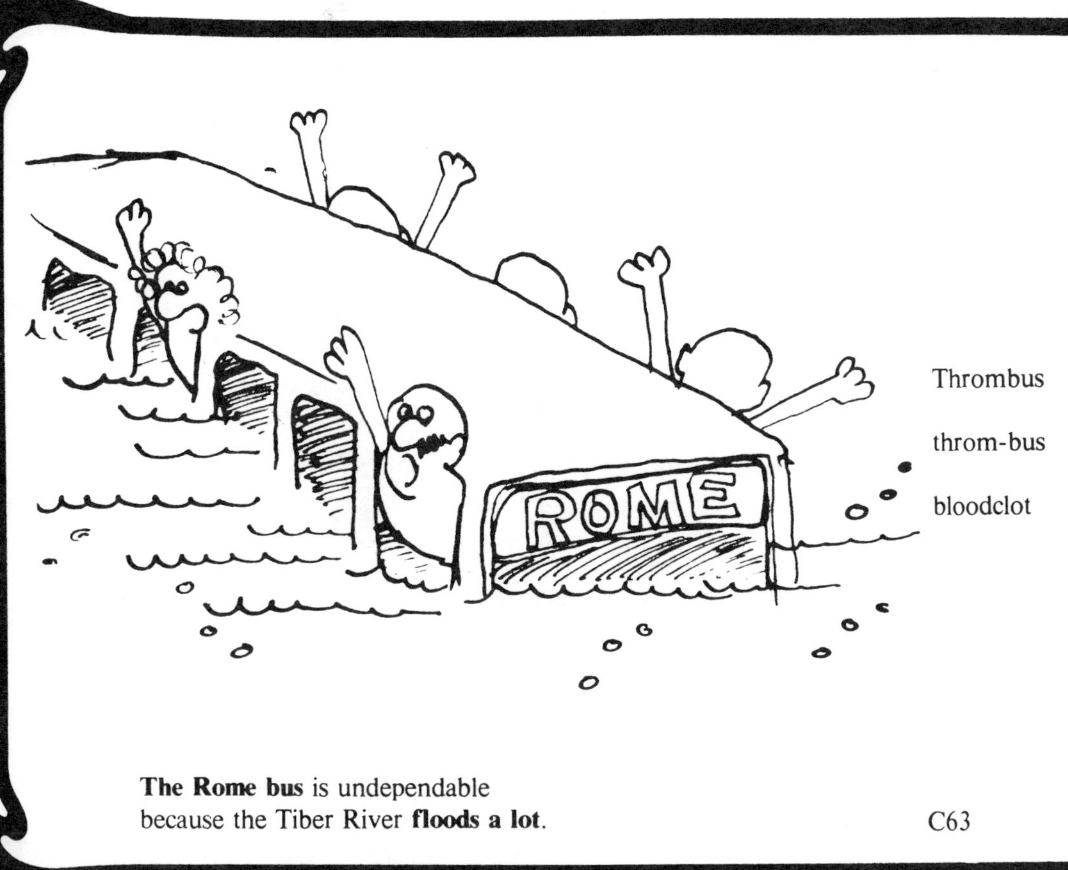

Thrombus

throm-bus

bloodclot

The Rome bus is undependable
because the Tiber River **floods a lot**.

C63

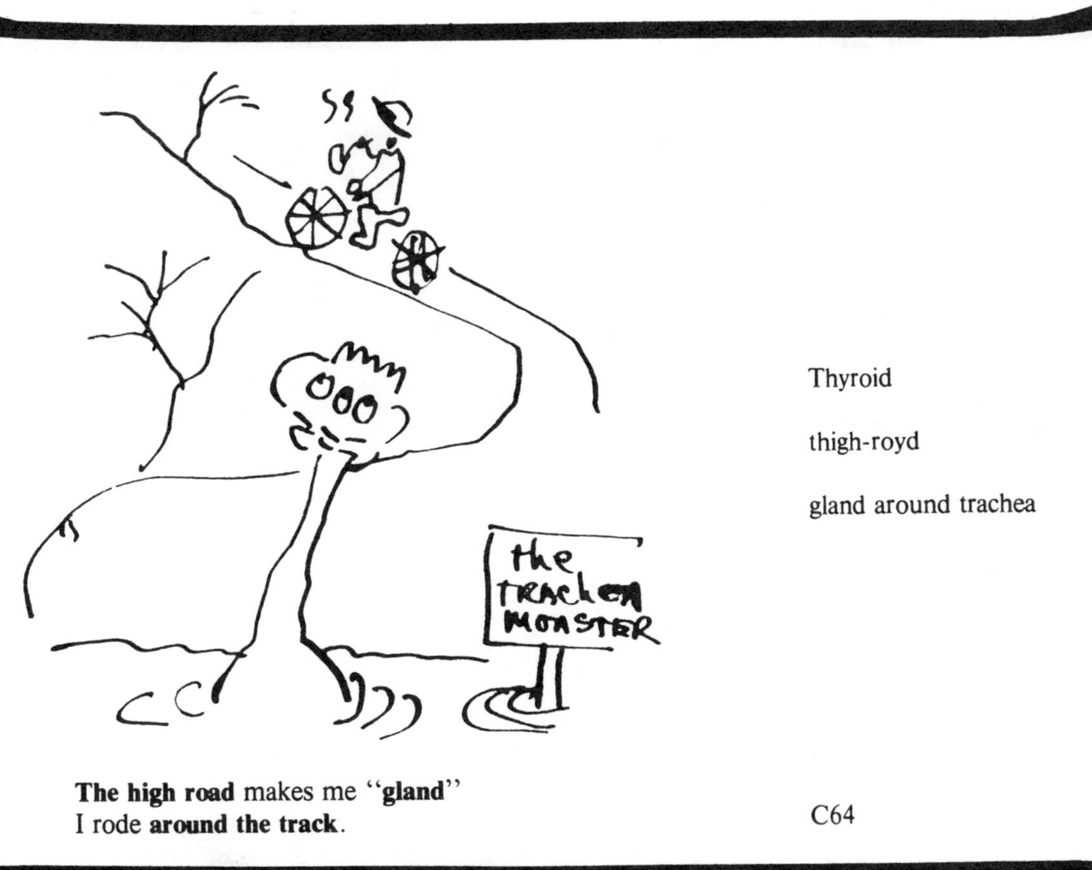

Thyroid

thigh-royd

gland around trachea

The high road makes me "**gland**"
I rode **around the track**.

C64

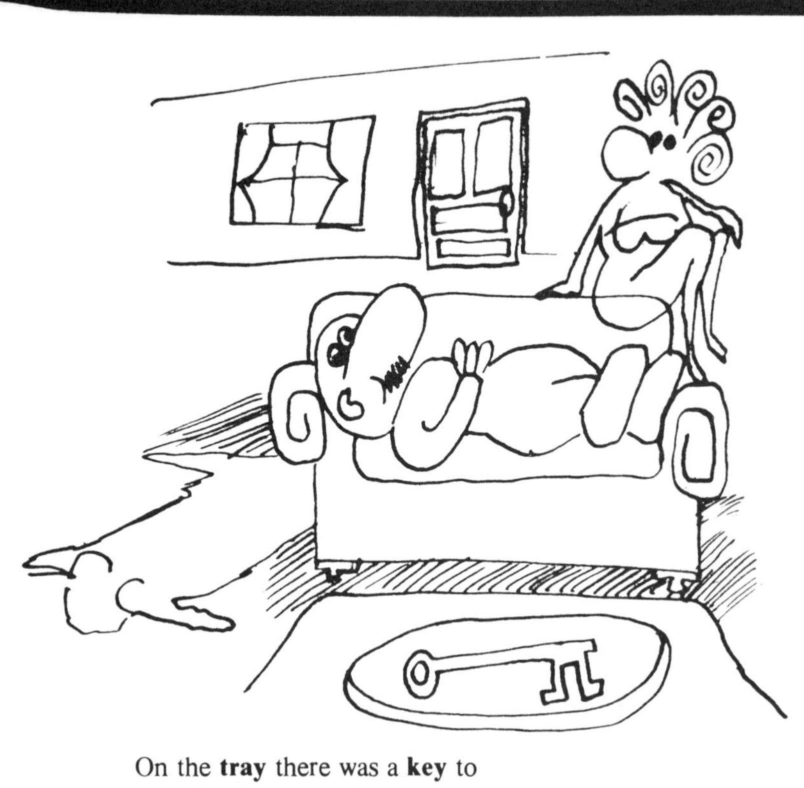

Trachea

tray-key-ah

tube between mouth
and lungs

On the **tray** there was a **key** to
open the **house** we **lounge** in.

C65

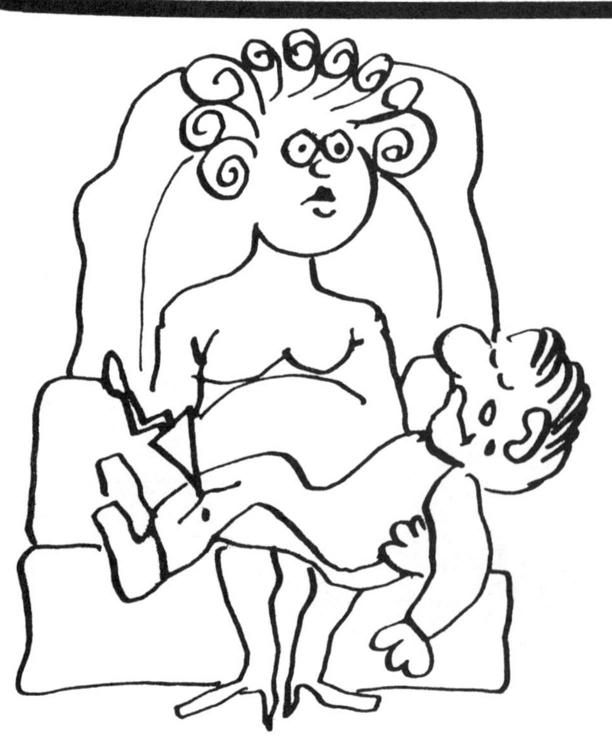

Trauma

traw-ma

injury

If you **injure** yourself with a
trowel, Ma will comfort you.

C66

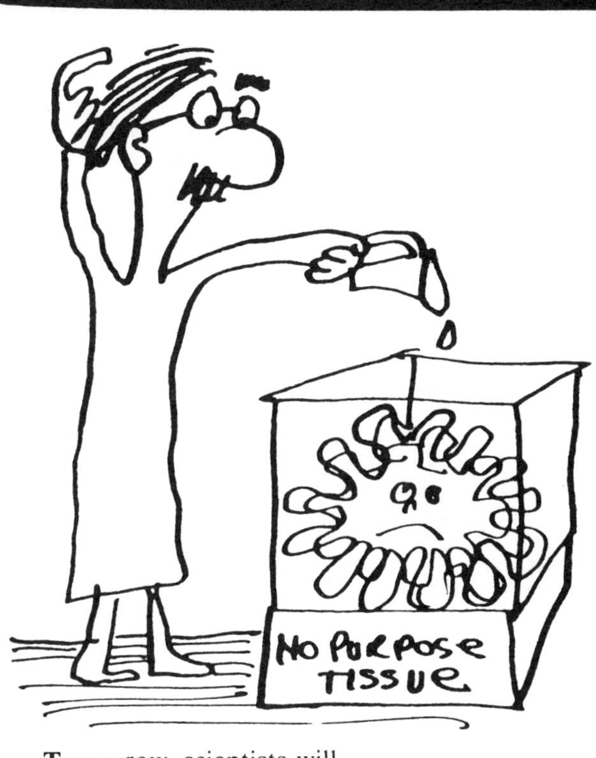

Tomorrow, scientists will
grow tissues with no purpose.

Tumor

two-more

growth of tissue
with no purpose

C67

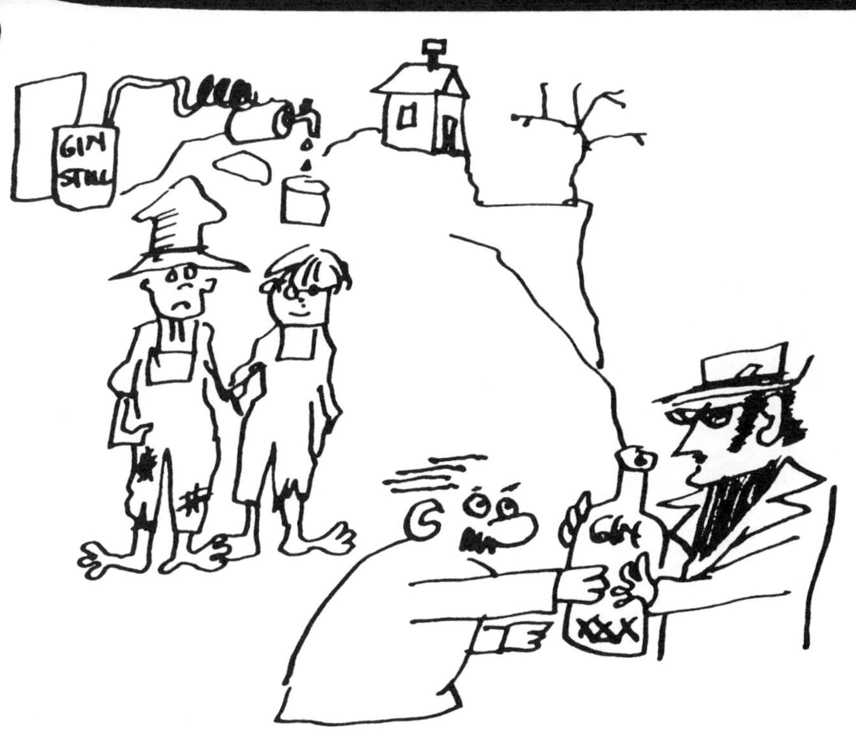

You're a terrible person to be **carrying
gin from the kids to the "blad" guys**.

Ureter

you-reh-ter

tube carrying urine
from kidney to bladder

C68

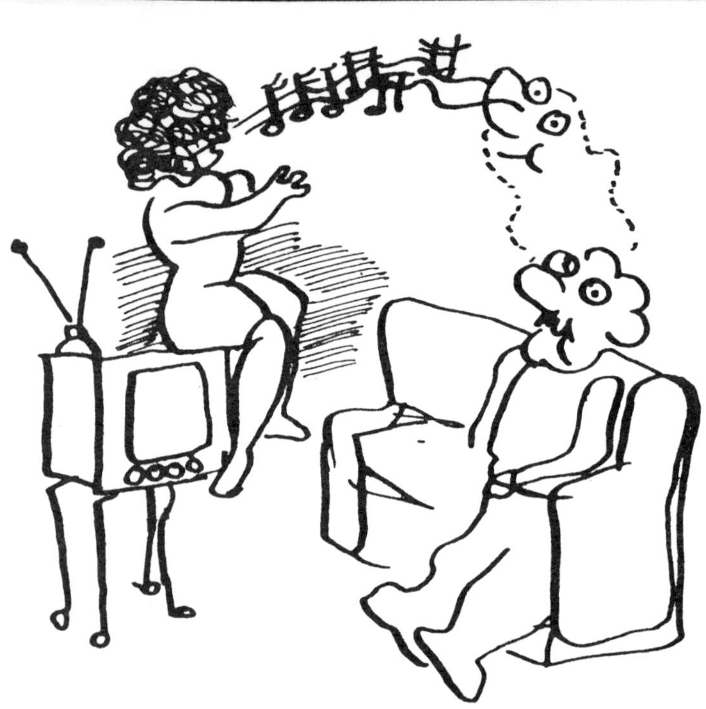

When **Urethra** is on the **tube,** she
carries the mood **you're in outside your body.**

Urethra

your-eeth-rah

tube that carries urine
outside body

C69

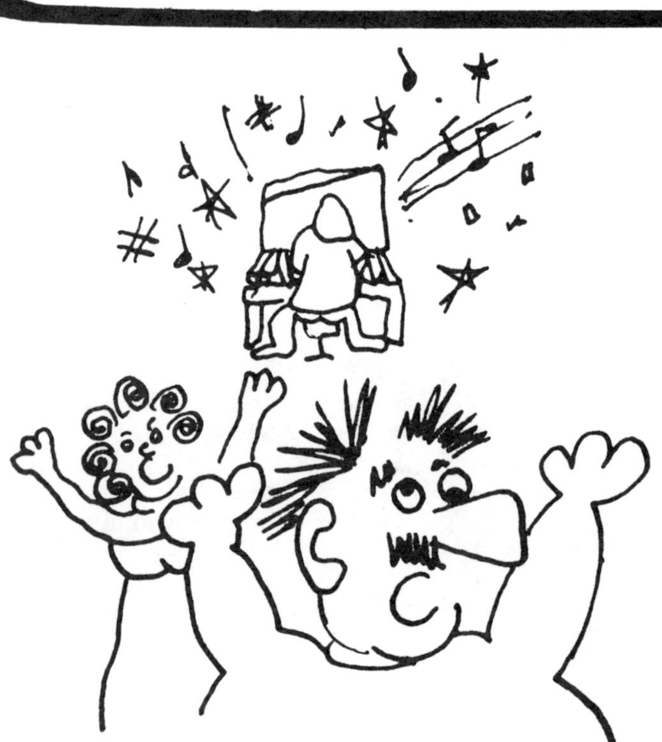

You're dear to us but you're not
whom we want to **organ**ize the party.

Uterus

you-der-us

female reproductive
organ; womb

C70

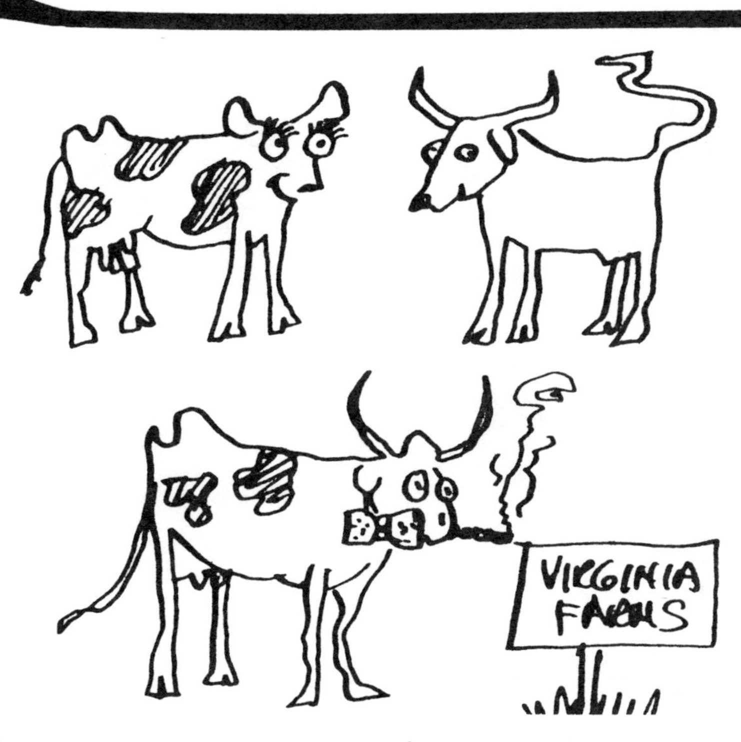

In **Virginia** were **born calves** of both **sexes** and **in the course** of time steers began to appear.

Vagina

va-jai-nah

birth cavity; female organ of sexual intercourse

C71

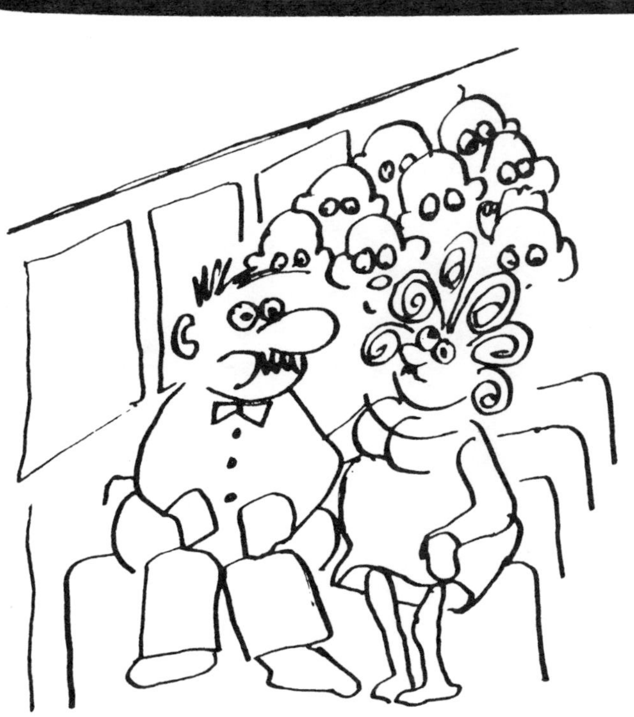

Vhen trollies ran, everybody **sure faced front** and not back.

Ventral

ven-trahl

front surface of the body

C72

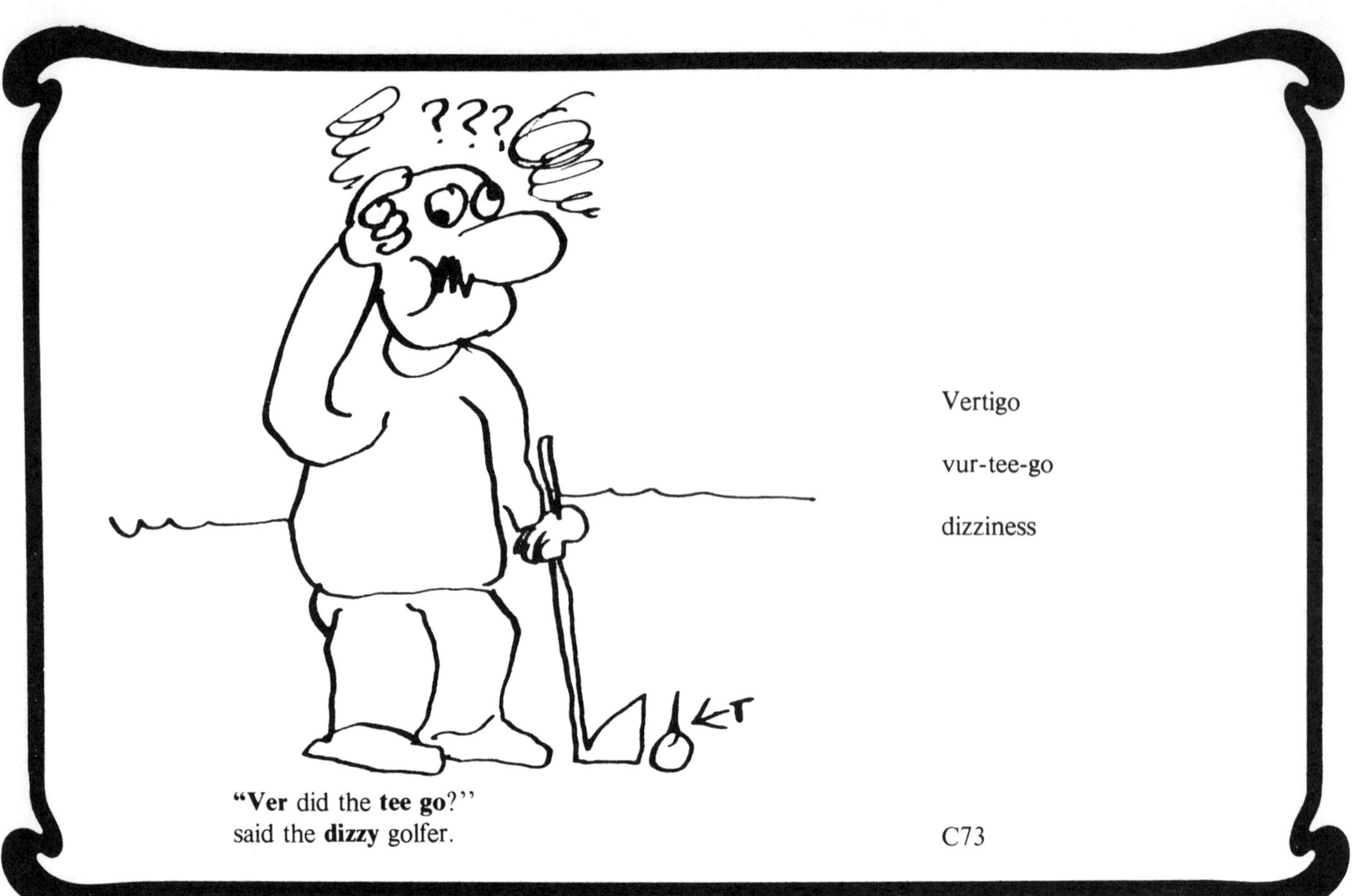

"Ver did the **tee go**?''
said the **dizzy** golfer.

Vertigo

vur-tee-go

dizziness

C73

WORD/PICTURE ASSOCIATIONS

SUFFIXES D

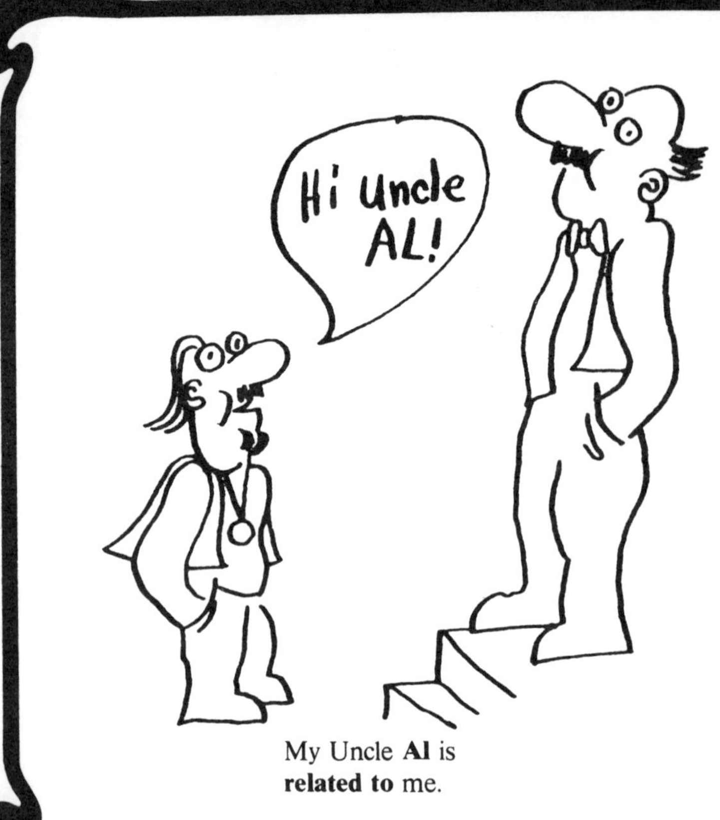

My Uncle **Al** is
related to me.

-Al

all

related to

D1

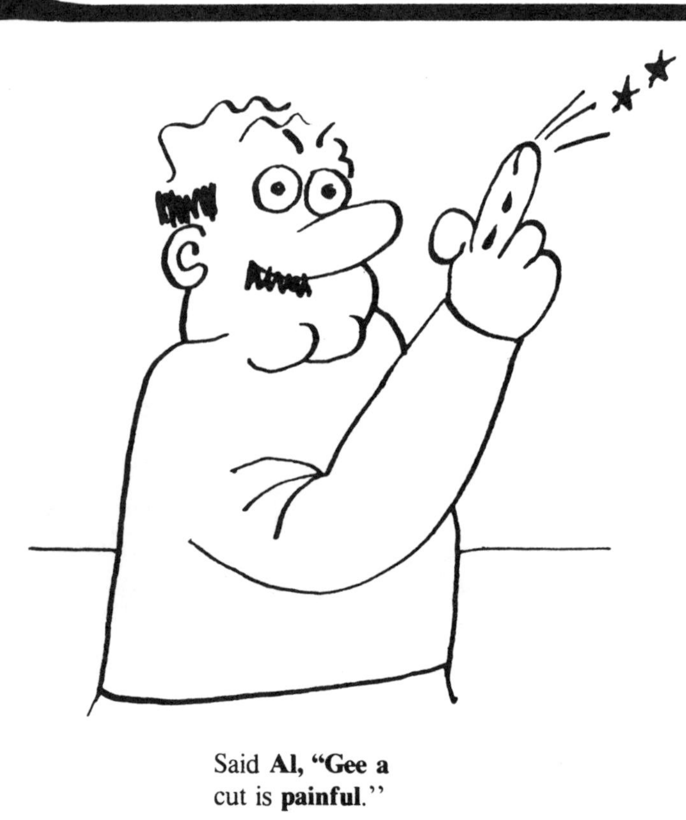

Said **Al**, "**Gee a**
cut is **painful**."

-Algia

al-ja

painful

D2

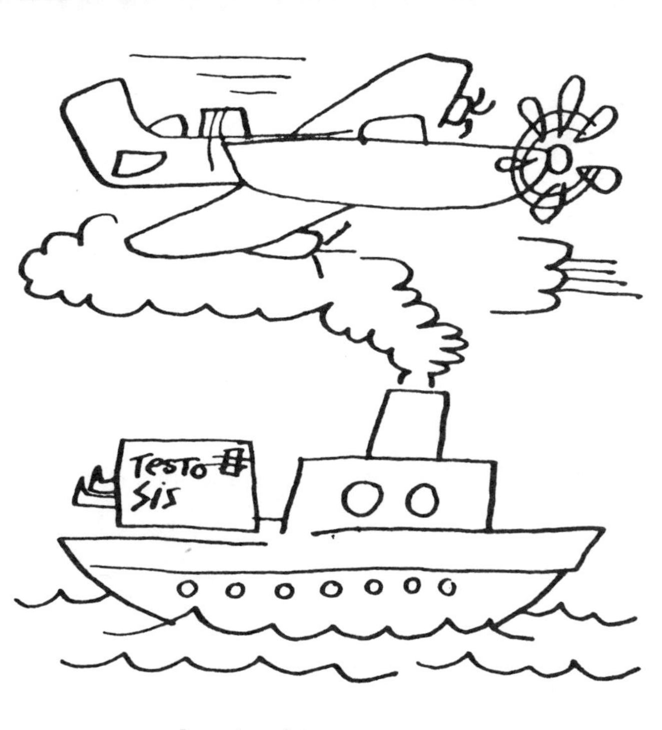

-Centesis

cen-ta-sis

to puncture; to let
out air or fluid

I **sent a si**ster to
puncture the tire.

D3

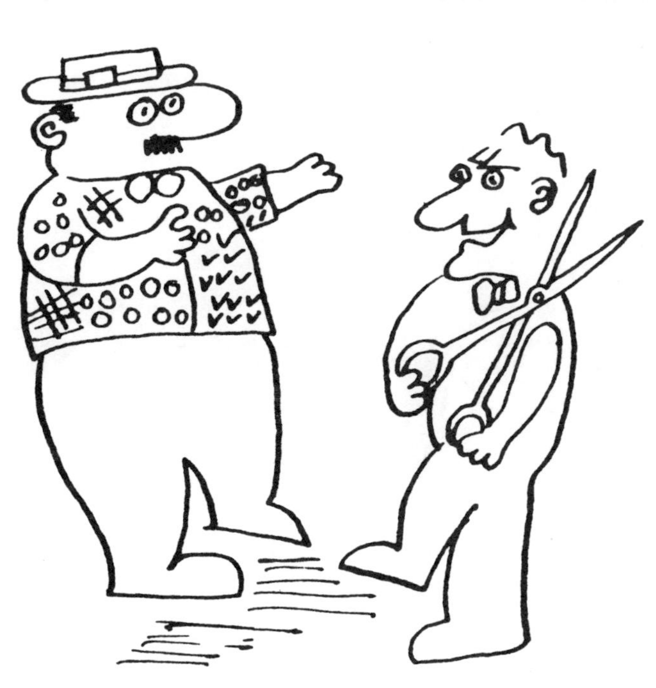

-Ectomy

eck-ta-mee

remove surgically

Cut it out, give
the **check to me**.

D4

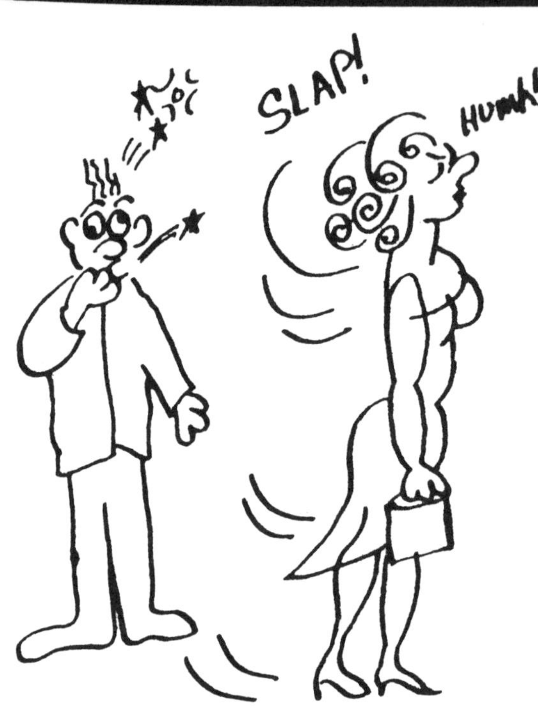

Young men with no sisters often have
no **knowledge of** a woman's **condition.**

-Gnosis

no-siss

knowledge of condition

D5

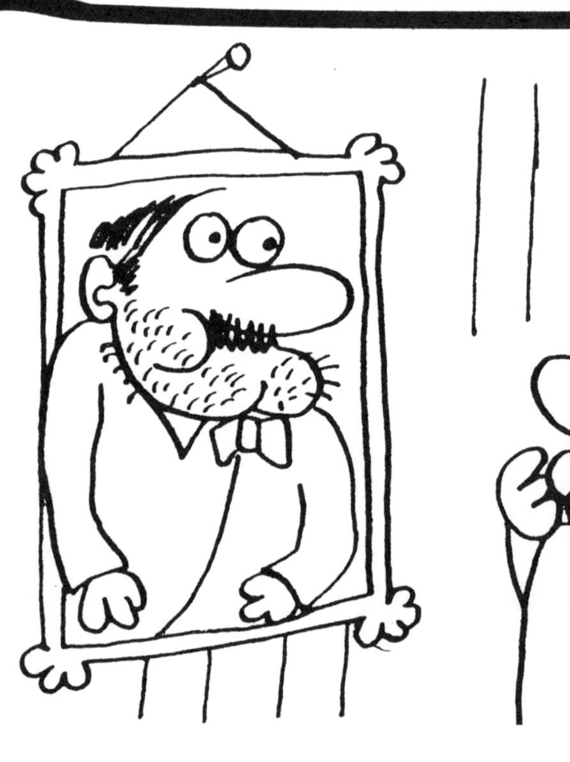

If you don't shave, any **picture
of** you will look **gruffy**.

-Graphy

gruf-fie

a picture of

D6

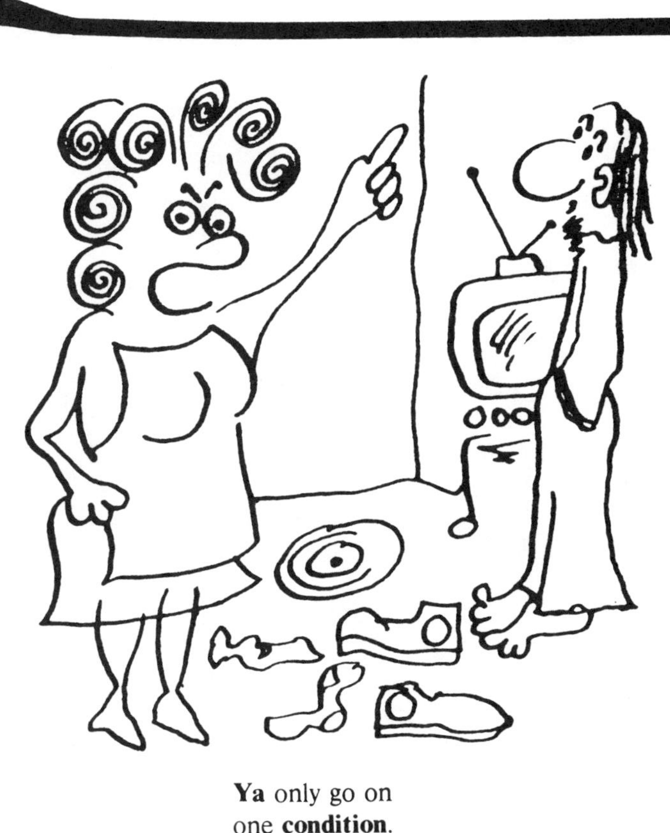

Ya only go on
one **condition**.

D7

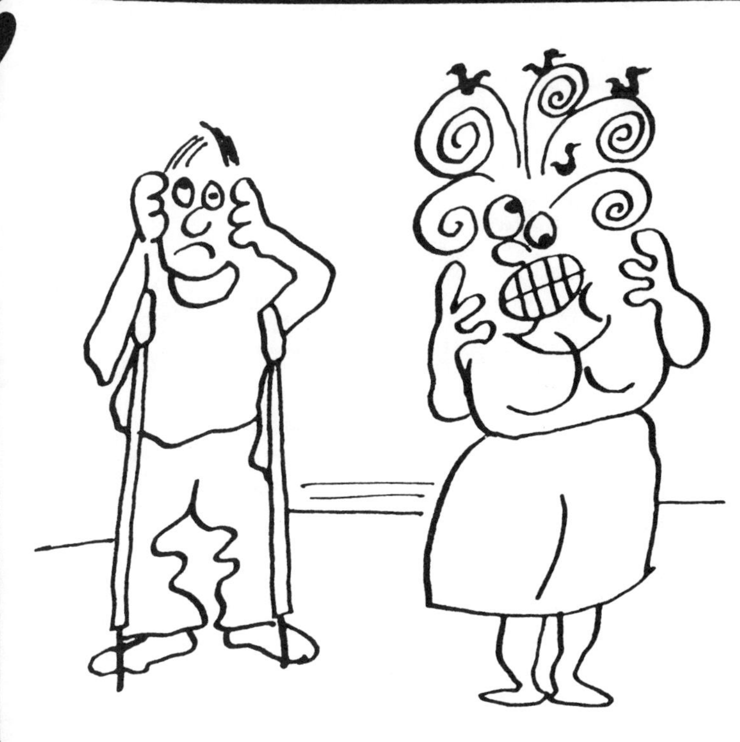

My **sick** uncle is **related
to** my crazy aunt.

D8

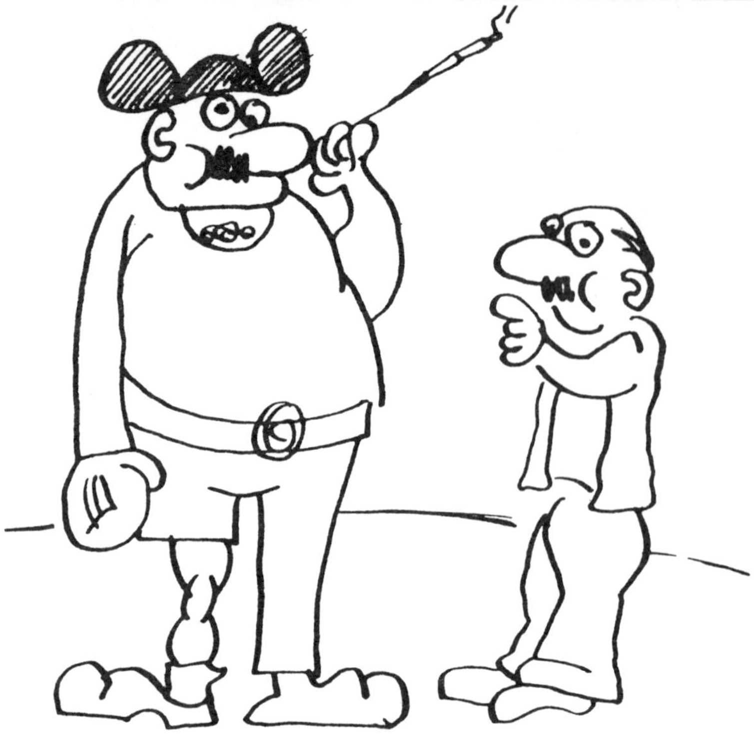

-Ism

iz-im

character of

Is my friend
a **character?**

D9

-Itis

eye-tiss

inflammation of

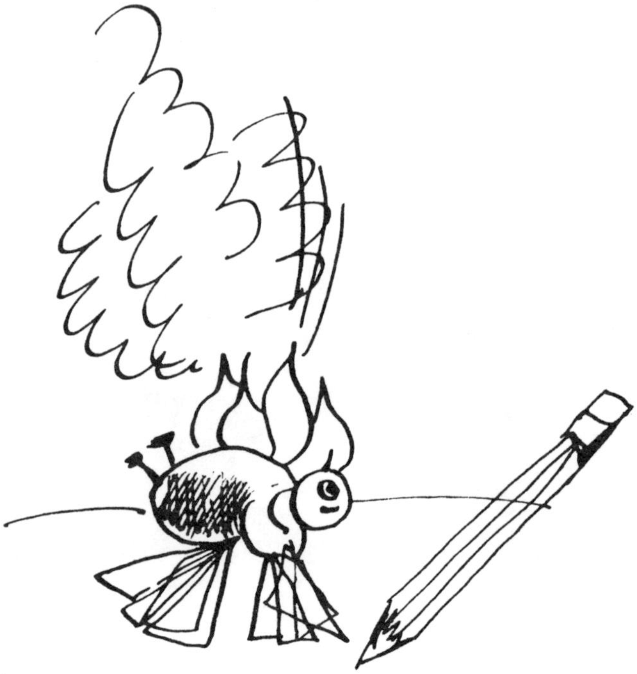

A **fly tiss** dead
when **in flames**.

D10

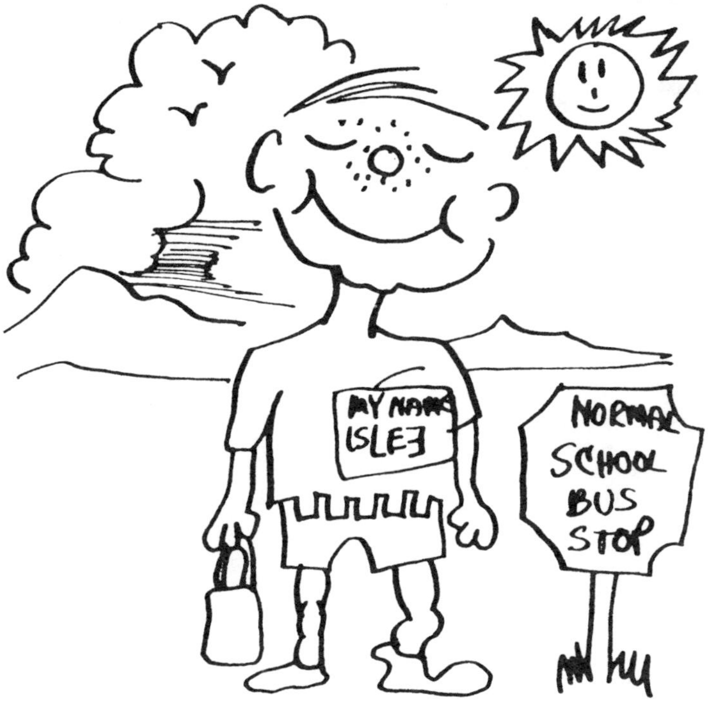

-Nomaly

nom-a-lee

normal

A **name** **like Lee** is
normal for a boy.

D11

-Norexia

no-rex-ya

appetite

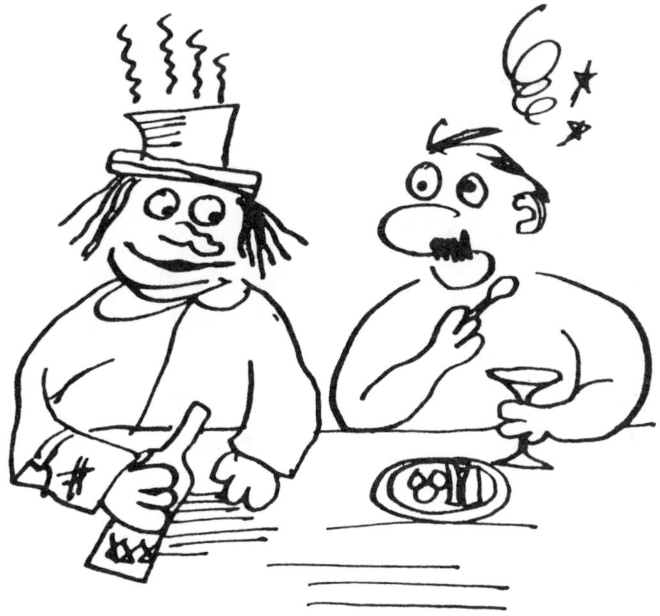

No, Rex! Ya make
me lose my **appetite**.

D12

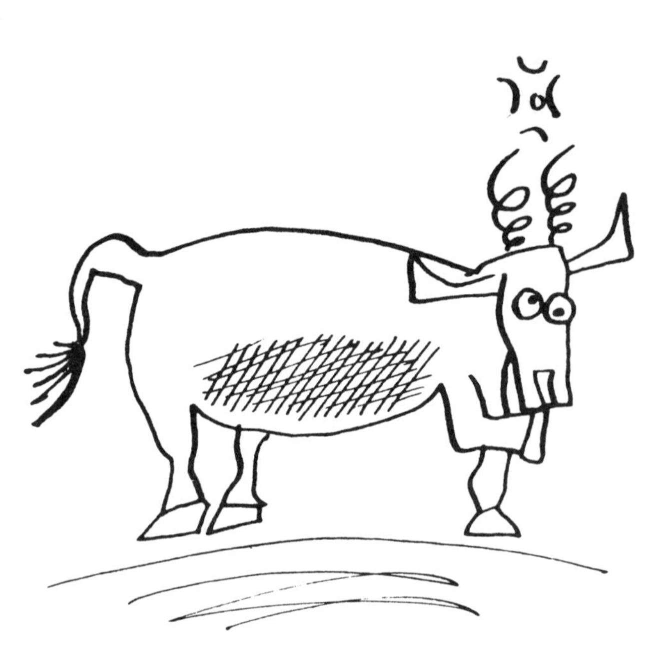

-Noxia

nox-ee-ah

oxygen

An ox, he has poor **oxygen**
if he works too hard.

D13

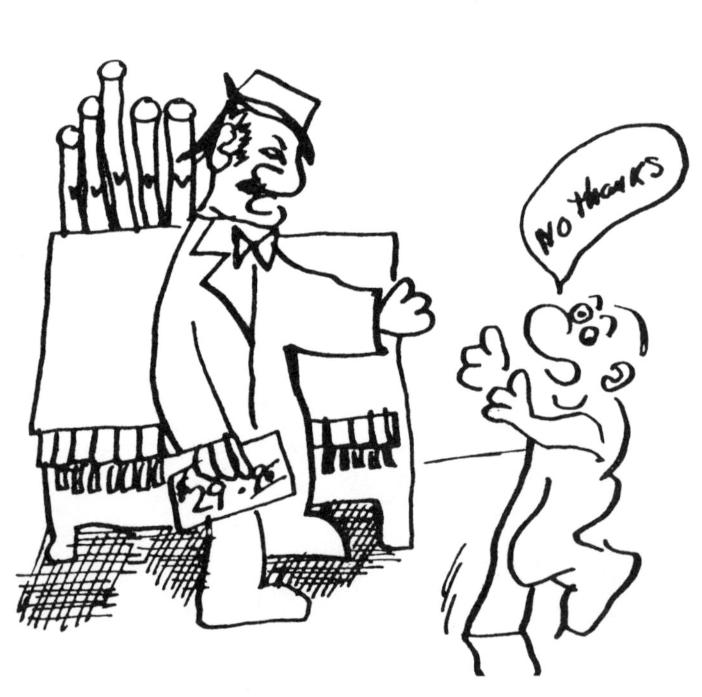

-Ocele

o-seal

sticking out
of an organ

No seal or price tag **sticks out
of an organ** bought in a good store.

D14

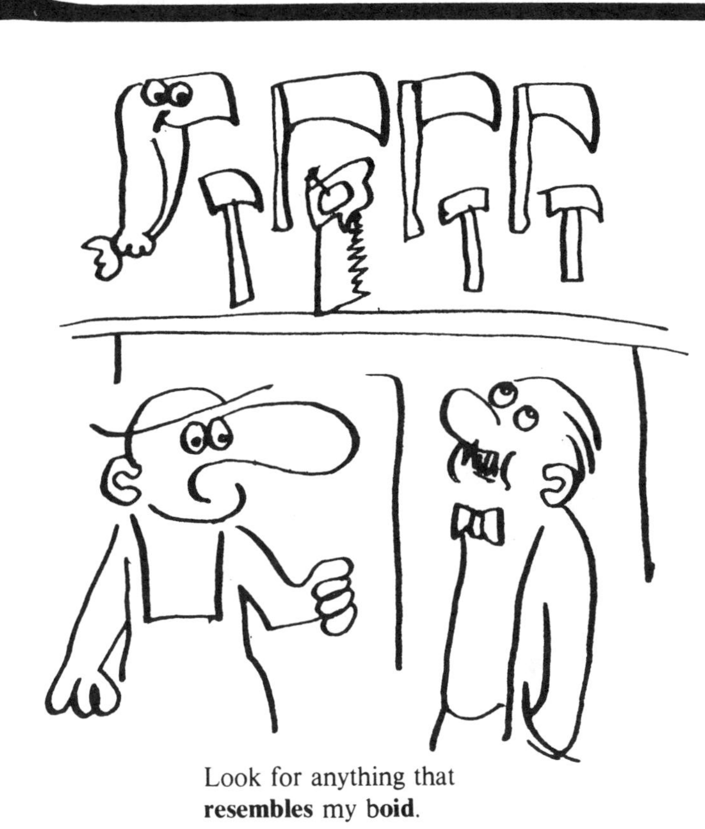

-Oid

oyd

resemble

D15

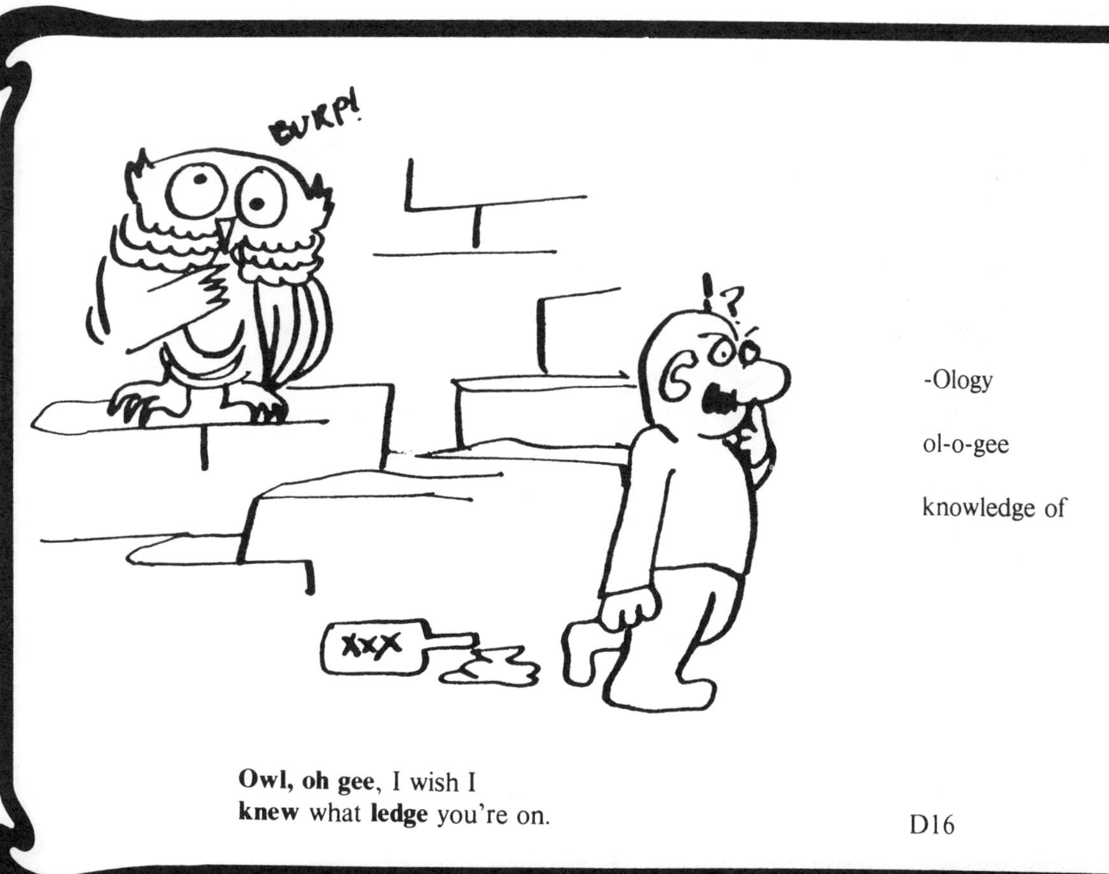

Owl, oh gee, I wish I
knew what **ledge** you're on.

-Ology

ol-o-gee

knowledge of

D16

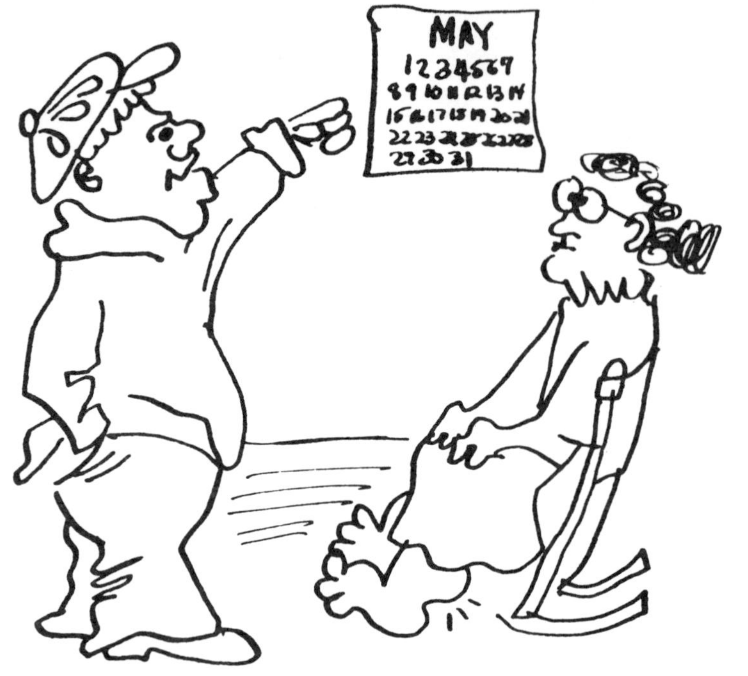

Last day **o'May**
is **tomor**row.

-Oma

o-ma

tumor

D17

Fid**o's paws ceased**
their scratching.

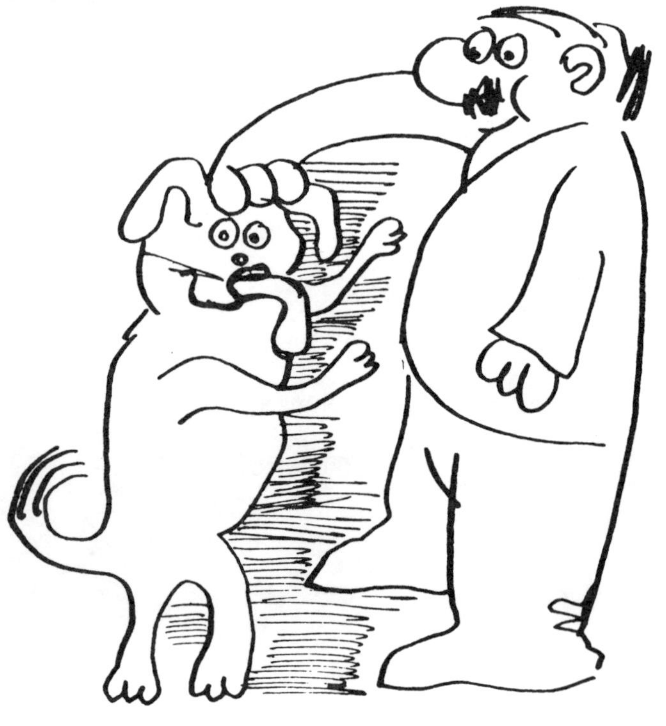

-Opause

o-paws

cessation; stoppage

D18

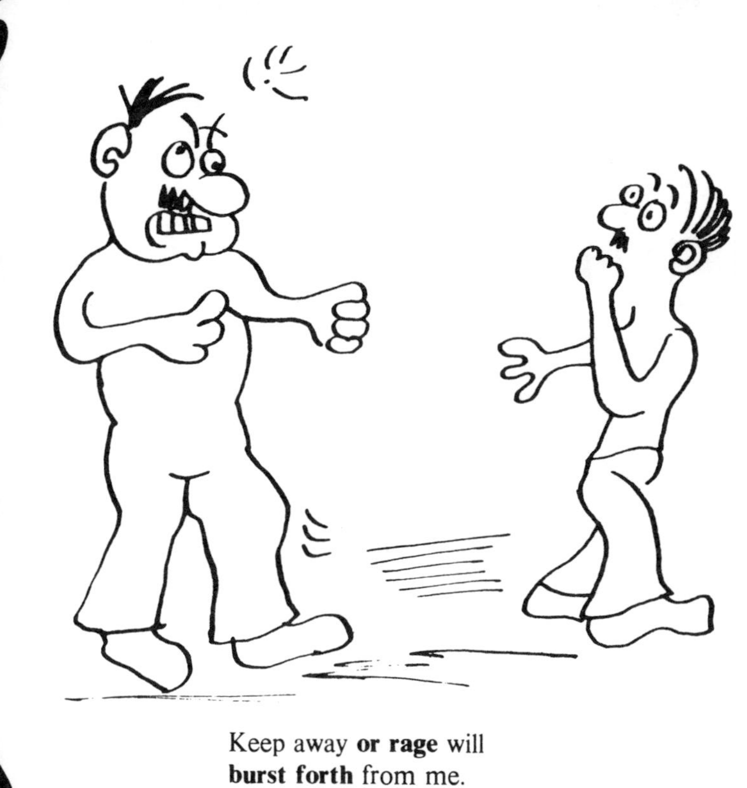

-Orrhage/-Orrhea

or-hage/o-re-a

burst forth

D19

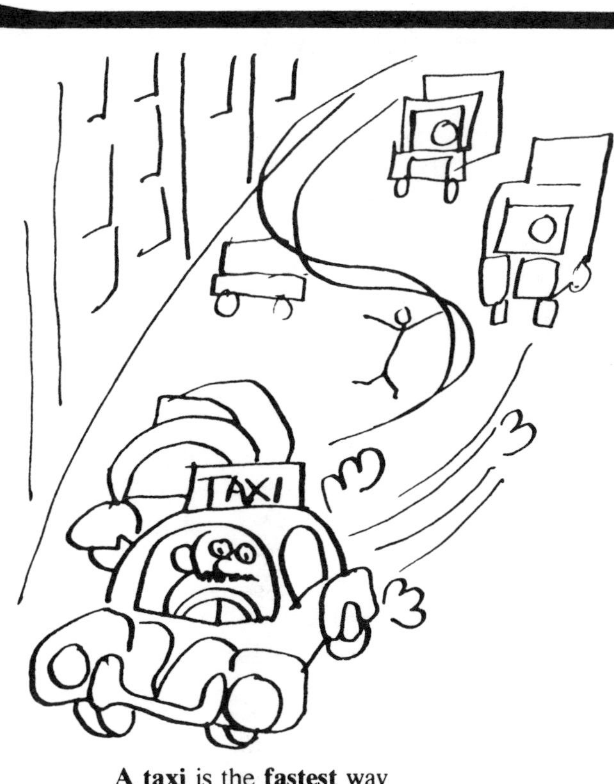

A taxi is the **fastest** way
to **surge** through the town.

-Pexy

pex-ee

to fasten surgically

D20

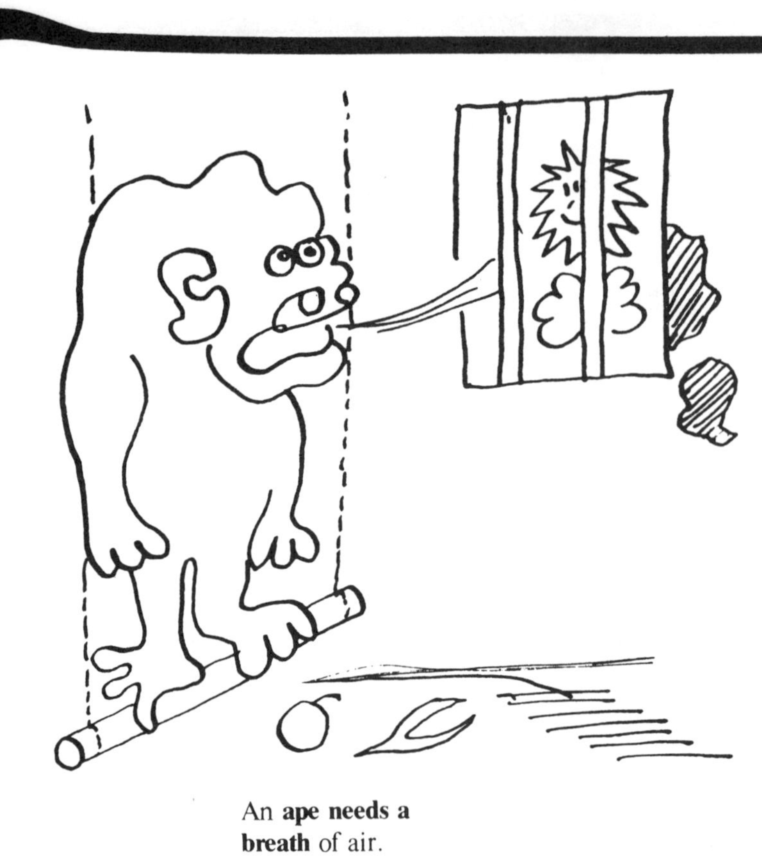

-Pnea

p-nee-a

breath

An **ape needs a breath** of air.

D21

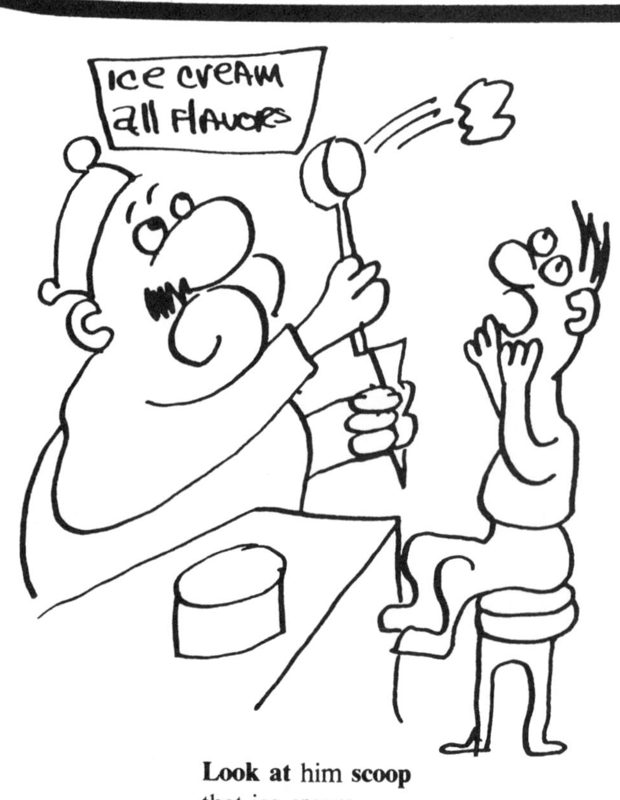

-Scope/-Scopy

skope: instrument used
to examine or
look at
skopy: to examine

Look at him **scoop** that ice cream.

D22

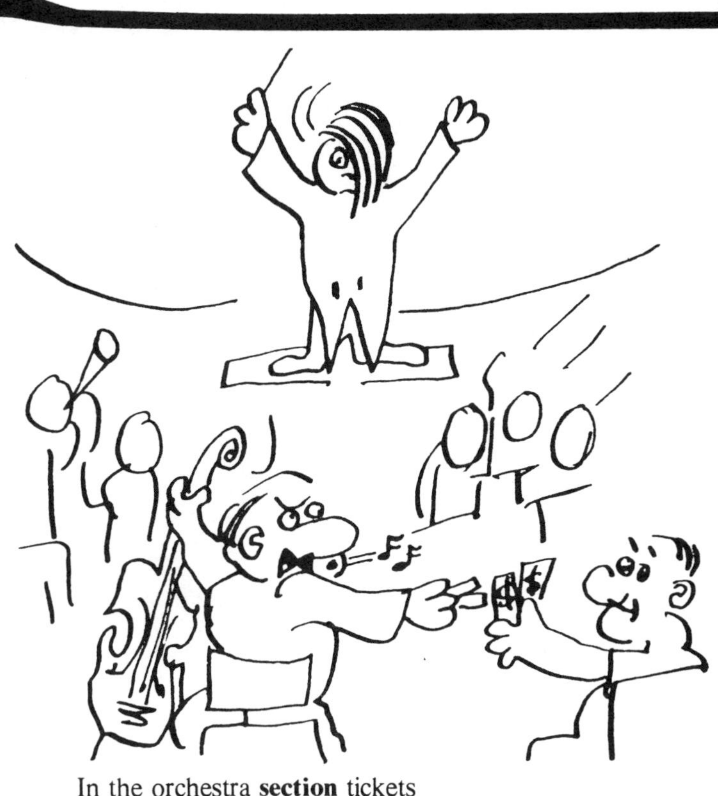

In the orchestra **section** tickets
were **issued** for the next **organ** concert.

Section

seck-shun

tissue or organ

D23

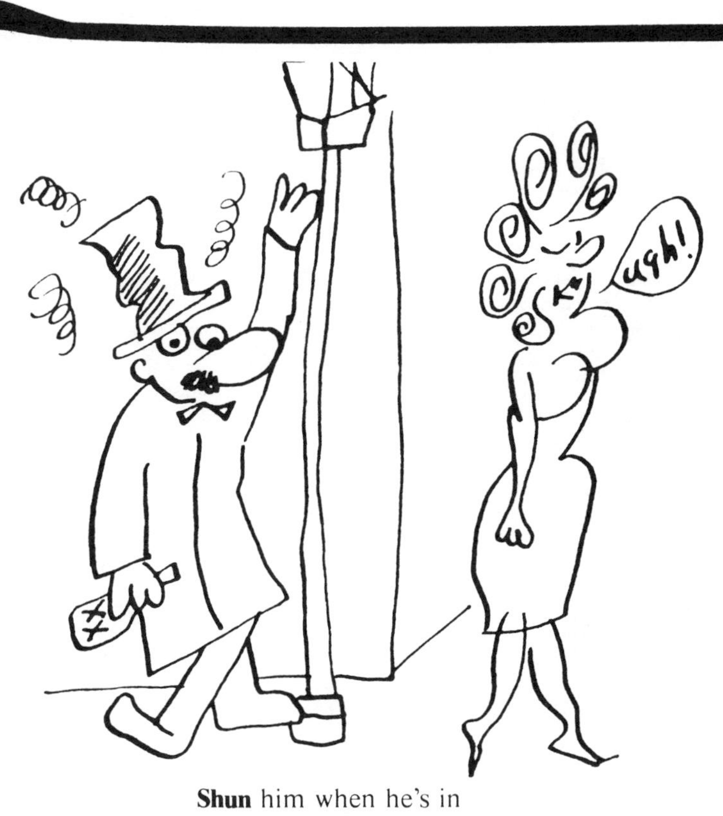

Shun him when he's in
a drunken **condition.**

-Sion/-Tion

shun

condition of being

D24

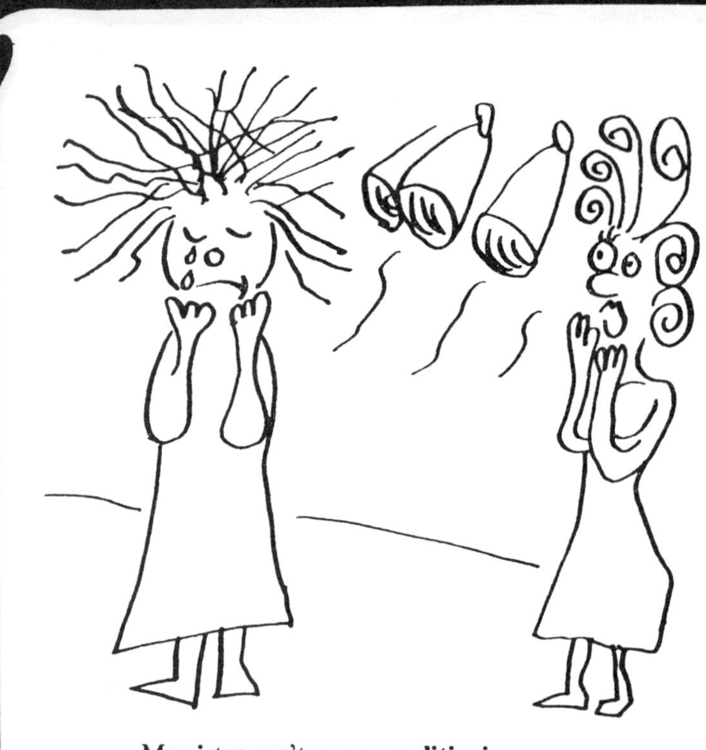

My **sister** can't use a **conditioning process** on her hair.

-Sis

siss

process; condition

D25

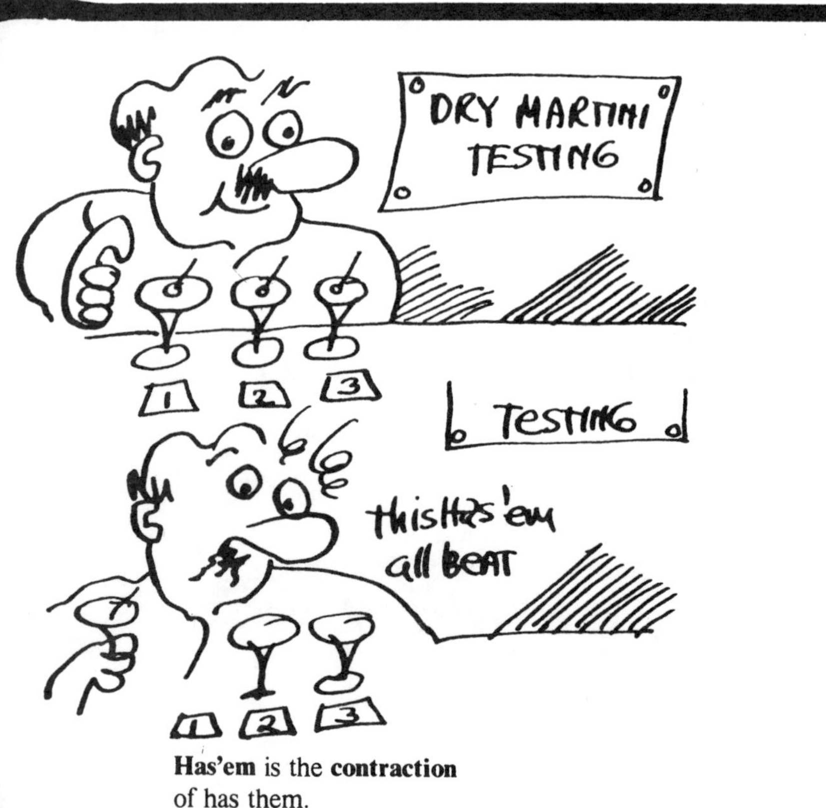

Has'em is the **contraction** of has them.

-Spasm

spaz-um

contraction of;
a cramp

D26

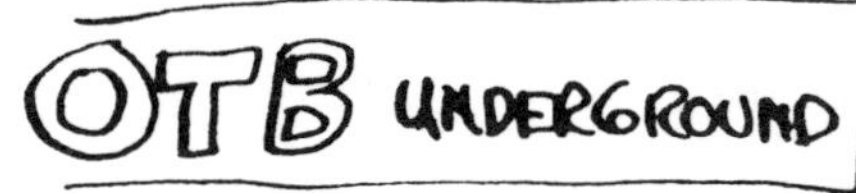

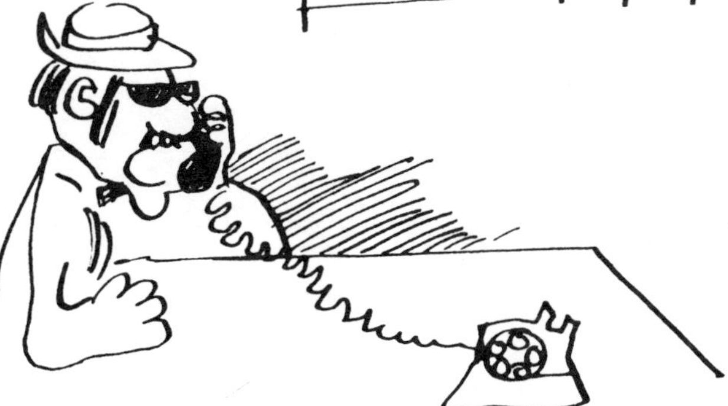

-Tomy/-Stomy

(also -Otomy)

(o) t-a-mee

to cut; make a
permanent opening

Don't **cut** off the phone **to me;**
I have a **permanent open** line.

D27

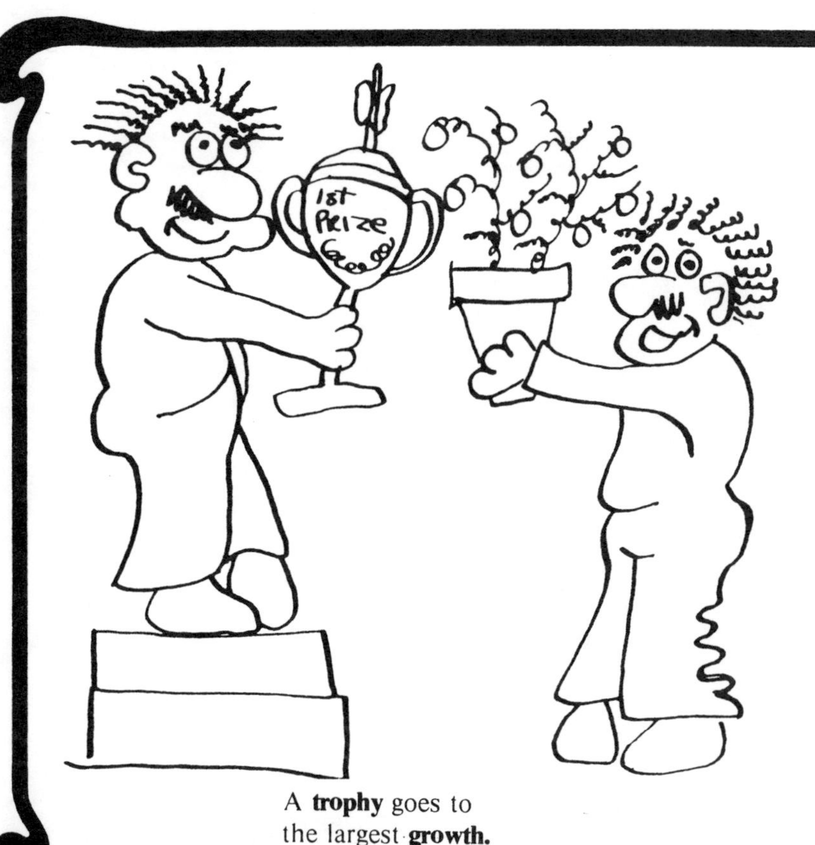

-Trophy

tro-fee

growth

A **trophy** goes to
the largest **growth.**

D28

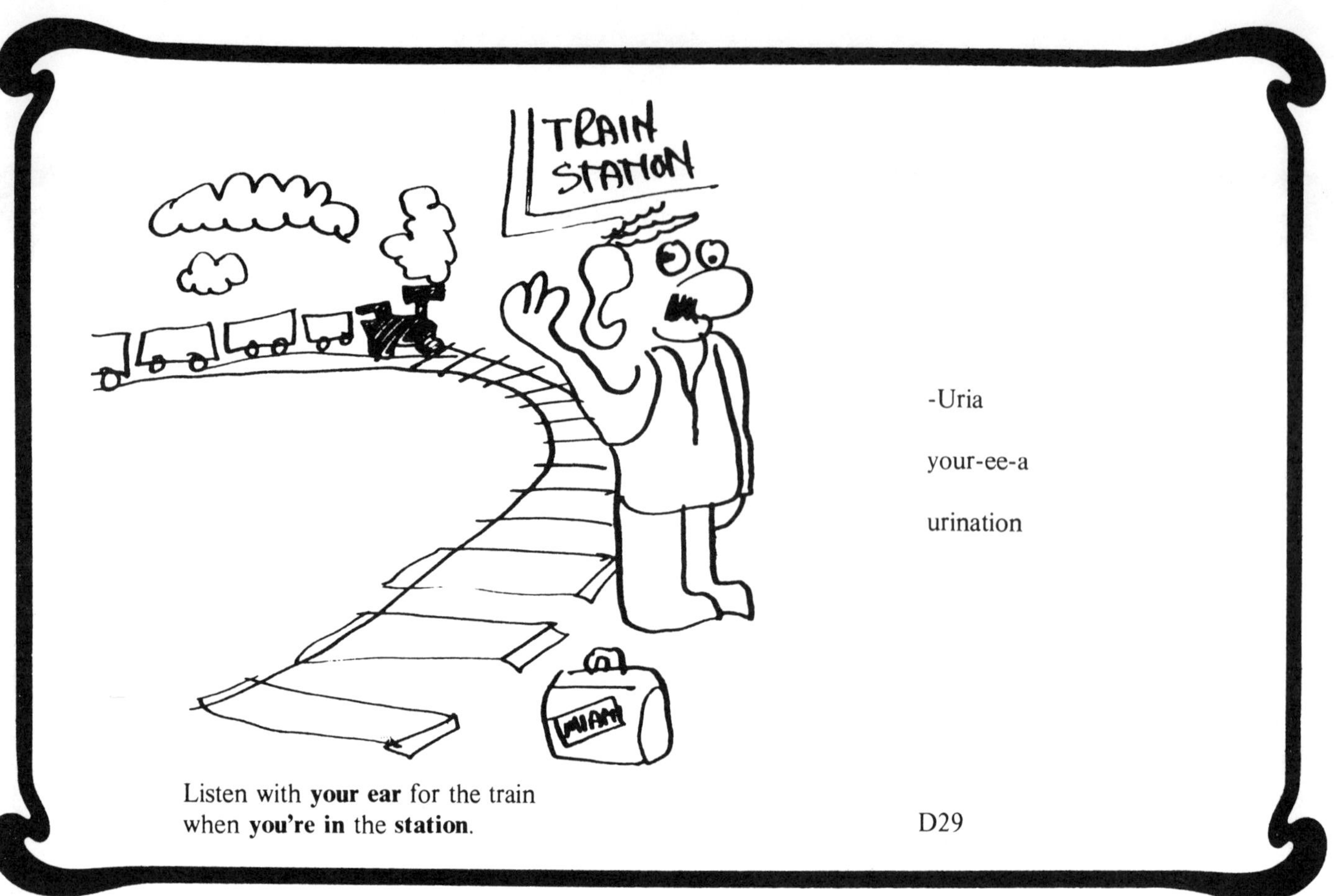

Listen with **your ear** for the train
when **you're in** the station.

-Uria

your-ee-a

urination

D29

EXERCISES

MATCHING
TRUE/FALSE
FILL-IN-THE-BLANKS

Instructions--Matching Exercises

The following matching exercises include all the prefixes and suffixes you have encountered in the 202 index words. Additionally, those 202 words are repeated here as a separate exercise.

This time, however, instead of selecting the one right answer out of the four choices given, you are presented with the words (or prefixes and suffixes) in groups of twelve, with the corresponding correct definitions for those twelve words listed along side, but not in the correct order. You are to match the correct definition (lettered A through J) with the numbered word and write the letter in the blank next to the word, as shown in the following example:

1. _C_ oak   A. a color
2. _A_ red   B. an animal
3. _B_ tiger   C. a tree

Follow this same procedure for all three matching exercises.

The answers for the prefix and suffix matching exercises are found on page 152, and answers for the whole word exercise are on page 153. Mark all incorrect answers with an X, and again study these words by referring to their corresponding Word/Picture Associations.

Prefix Multiple Choice

1. _____ a-
2. _____ aden-
3. _____ adhe-
4. _____ anastomo-
5. _____ aneury-
6. _____ angio-
7. _____ arthr-
8. _____ brady-
9. _____ carcin-
10. _____ cardi(a)-
11. _____ cauteriza-
12. _____ chole-

A. blood vessel
B. burn tissue
C. not; without; lessen
D. malignant
E. gall
F. join two parts to make a new passageway
G. gland; glandular tissue
H. ballooning out of blood vessel at a weak point
I. slow
J. abnormal sticking together
K. heart
L. joints

13. _____ chondri-
14. _____ chron-
15. _____ concus-
16. _____ congenit-
17. _____ contu-
18. _____ convul-
19. _____ coronary
20. _____ cyano-
21. _____ de-
22. _____ dermat-
23. _____ dia-
24. _____ dist-

A. existing at birth
B. slow down; decrease
C. cartilage
D. part of limb furthest away from the trunk
E. bruise
F. identification
G. jarring injury to the brain
H. long duration; recurring frequently
I. heart attack due to blocked coronary vessels
J. blue appearance of skin
K. irregular movements of limbs
L. skin

25. _____ dors-
26. _____ dys-
27. _____ dysmen-
28. _____ ectop-
29. _____ embol-
30. _____ en-
31. _____ endo-
32. _____ enter(o)-
33. _____ entop-
34. _____ excis-
35. _____ fibr-
36. _____ frozen

A. inside
B. difficulty; painful
C. rapid examination of tissue
D. inside
E. to occur outside or in an unusual place
F. remove by cutting out
G. occurring in a normal place
H. fibrous tissue
I. floating bloodclot blocking the vessel
J. back surface of the body
K. intestine
L. painful menses

37. _____ gall
38. _____ gastro-
39. _____ hem(at)-
40. _____ hemopty-
41. _____ hepat-
42. _____ hydro-
43. _____ hyper-
44. _____ hystero-
45. _____ intern-
46. _____ lacera-
47. _____ lapar-
48. _____ laryngo-

A. water
B. away from body surface
C. voice box
D. blood
E. uterus
F. bile
G. over; excessively
H. abdomen
I. stomach
J. spit blood from lungs
K. tear or cut in skin
L. liver

49. _____ loc-
50. _____ men-
51. _____ metasta-
52. _____ my-
53. _____ myelo-
54. _____ nephro-
55. _____ neuro-
56. _____ oophor-
57. _____ orchi(do)-
58. _____ oste-
59. _____ para-
60. _____ peri-

A. nerves
B. around
C. bone
D. monthly flow
E. kidney
F. limited to specific area of the body
G. testicle
H. disease shifting from one part of the body to another
I. organs alongside any cavity
J. ovary
K. spinal cord
L. muscle

61. _____ peripher-
62. _____ periton-
63. _____ pneumon-
64. _____ pro-
65. _____ procto-
66. _____ proxim-
67. _____ pto-
68. _____ system-
69. _____ tachy-
70. _____ tenon-
71. _____ un-
72. _____ vaso-
73. _____ ventila-

A. breathing
B. part of limb nearest trunk
C. forecast
D. lining inside of abdomen
E. fast
F. lung
G. outside of; external
H. none; not
I. vessel
J. tendon
K. rectum
L. entire body
M. drooping of an organ

Suffix Multiple Choice

1. ____ -al
2. ____ -algia
3. ____ -centesis
4. ____ -ectomy
5. ____ -gnosis
6. ____ -graphy
7. ____ -ia
8. ____ -ic
9. ____ -ism
10. ____ -itis

A. knowledge of condition
B. character of
C. remove surgically
D. painful
E. inflammation of
F. to puncture; to let out air or fluid
G. condition of
H. related to
I. picture of
J. related to

11. ____ -nomaly
12. ____ -norexia
13. ____ -noxia
14. ____ -ocele
15. ____ -oid
16. ____ -ology
17. ____ -oma
18. ____ -opause
19. ____ -orrhage/-orrhea
20. ____ -pexy

A. knowledge of
B. normal
C. to fasten surgically
D. cessation; stoppage
E. tumor
F. appetite
G. burst forth
H. sticking out of an organ
I. oxygen
J. resemble

21. ____ -pnea
22. ____ -scope/-scopy
23. ____ -section
24. ____ -sion/-tion
25. ____ -sis
26. ____ -spasm
27. ____ -(o)tomy/-stomy
28. ____ -trophy
29. ____ -uria

A. cut; make permanent opening
B. breath
C. contraction of; a cramp
D. process; condition
E. instrument used to examine or to look at; to examine
F. urination
G. tissue or organ
H. growth
I. condition of being

Whole Words Multiple Choice

1. ____ abdomen	A. glandular tissue tumors
2. ____ abdominal	B. rapid course and short duration
3. ____ abdominocentesis	C. join two parts together to make a new passageway
4. ____ acquired	D. relating to abdominal cavity
5. ____ acute	E. abnormal sticking together
6. ____ adenoid	F. abdominal puncture to let out air
7. ____ adenoma	G. entire breathing passage
8. ____ adhesion	H. gland-like
9. ____ airway	I. shock occurring after injection of drug because of allergy to drug
10. ____ anaphylactic shock	J. cavity containing stomach
11. ____ anastomosis	K. ballooning out of blood vessel
12. ____ aneurysm	L. developed after birth

13. ____ angiography	A. painful joints
14. ____ angiospasm	B. shortage of oxygen
15. ____ anomaly	C. paralysis and fainting due to stroke
16. ____ anorexia	D. vessel cramp
17. ____ anoxia	E. inflammation of joints
18. ____ anus	F. loss of appetite
19. ____ apnea	G. removal of appendix
20. ____ apoplexy	H. picture of blood vessels
21. ____ appendectomy	I. sac off large intestine
22. ____ appendix	J. opening at end of digestive tract
23. ____ arthralgia	K. temporary stoppage of breathing
24. ____ arthritis	L. vary from normal

25. ____ ascites	A. removal of tissue for microscopic examination
26. ____ aseptic	B. malignant tumor
27. ____ atrophy	C. mild and not recurring
28. ____ benign	D. to look inside bronchi
29. ____ biopsy	E. free of pus-producing germs
30. ____ bladder	F. a stone
31. ____ bradycardia	G. fluid in abdominal cavity
32. ____ bronchi	H. slow heartbeat
33. ____ bronchial endoscope	I. wasting away of body parts
34. ____ bronchoscopy	J. right and left windpipes which enter lungs
35. ____ calculus	K. sac-like structure collecting urine
36. ____ cancer	L. examination of bronchi with a special instrument

37. _____ carcinoma
38. _____ cardiac arrest
39. _____ cardiology
40. _____ cauterization
41. _____ cephalgia
42. _____ cephalic
43. _____ cephalus
44. _____ cerebral
45. _____ cerebral hemorrhage
46. _____ cerebrum
47. _____ cholecystectomy
48. _____ cholelithiasis

A. malignant tumor
B. bursting of brain blood vessel
C. relating to the head
D. relating to the brain
E. headache
F. removal of the gall bladder
G. the study of the heart
H. formation of gall stones
I. destroy tissue by burning
J. the brain
K. stoppage of the heart
L. the head

49. _____ chondritis
50. _____ chronic
51. _____ clean
52. _____ colon
53. _____ colostomy
54. _____ coma
55. _____ concussion
56. _____ congenital
57. _____ contusion
58. _____ convulsion
59. _____ coronary thrombosis
60. _____ cranial

A. large intestine
B. irregular body movements
C. deep unconsciousness
D. heart attack due to clot in coronary vessels
E. free of pus-producing germs
F. existing at birth
G. inflammation of cartilage
H. relating to the skull
I. operation to make permanent hole in large intestine
J. injury to the brain
K. recurring frequently
L. bruise

61. _____ cranium
62. _____ craniotomy
63. _____ cyanosis
64. _____ cyst
65. _____ cystocele
66. _____ cystoscopy
67. _____ defibrillation
68. _____ dermatoid
69. _____ dermatoma
70. _____ diagnosis
71. _____ dirty
72. _____ disease

A. identification of condition
B. cutting the skull
C. sickness
D. protrusion of the bladder
E. slow heartbeat electrically
F. the skull
G. containing pus-producing germs
H. instrument examination of bladder
I. resembling skin
J. blue appearance of skin due to anoxia
K. skin tumor
L. bladder-like sac containing fluid

73. _____ distal
74. _____ dorsal
75. _____ dysmenorrhea
76. _____ dyspnea
77. _____ dysuria
78. _____ eclampsia
79. _____ ectopic
80. _____ edema
81. _____ embolism
82. _____ encephalography
83. _____ endotracheal
84. _____ enteritis

A. relating to inside of trachea
B. part of limb furthest from trunk
C. fluid in the tissue
D. painful flow of monthly menses
E. inflammation of intestine
F. convulsion before or after childbirth
G. a picture showing inside of head
H. difficulty breathing due to blocked airway
I. occurring outside the body
J. painful urination
K. blocking of vessel by traveling blood clot
L. back surface of body

85. _____ enterostomy
86. _____ entopic
87. _____ epistaxia
88. _____ esophageal endoscope
89. _____ esophagoscopy
90. _____ esophagus
91. _____ excision
92. _____ fibrillation
93. _____ fibroid
94. _____ fibroma
95. _____ fracture
96. _____ frozen section

A. examination of esophagus with an instrument
B. rapid examination of tissue
C. instrument used to look inside the esophagus
D. fast heartbeat
E. make permanent opening in intestine
F. fibrous tumor
G. tube from mouth to stomach
H. remove by cutting out
I. nosebleed
J. crack in bone
K. occurring in normal place
L. resembling fibrous tissue

97. _____ gall bladder
98. _____ gastralgia
99. _____ gastroenteritis
100. _____ heart
101. _____ hematology
102. _____ hemoptysis
103. _____ hemorrhage
104. _____ hepatitis
105. _____ hernia
106. _____ hydrocele
107. _____ hydroencephalograph
108. _____ hypertrophy

A. sac that stores bile
B. protrusion of an organ through wall or cavity
C. study of the blood
D. bursting forth of blood
E. painful stomach
F. inflammation of the liver
G. inflammation of stomach and intestine
H. water hernia in testicle
I. bleeding from lungs
J. excessive growth of body parts
K. muscular organ between lungs
L. picture of water inside head

109. _____ hyperventilation
110. _____ hysteropexy
111. _____ hysterotomy
112. _____ ileostomy
113. _____ ileum
114. _____ internal
115. _____ intestine
116. _____ kidney
117. _____ laceration
118. _____ laparotomy
119. _____ laryngospasm
120. _____ lesion

A. muscle contraction of voice box
B. overbreathing
C. organ manufacturing urine
D. fastening of uterus in place
E. area of diseased tissue
F. small intestine
G. tear in skin
H. cutting to make permanent opening in small intestine
I. lower digestive tract
J. the part of the body away from the surface
K. to cut into the abdomen
L. cutting of uterus

121. _____ liver
122. _____ local
123. _____ lungs
124. _____ malaise
125. _____ malignant
126. _____ meninges
127. _____ meningitis
128. _____ meningocele
129. _____ menopause
130. _____ menorrhagia
131. _____ metastasis
132. _____ metastatic

A. vague feeling of illness
B. herniation of brain covering
C. specific area of body
D. stoppage of monthly menses flow
E. brain covering
F. the shifting of disease from one part of the body to another
G. balloon-like structures in chest
H. inflammation of brain covering
I. organ producing bile
J. excessive menstrual flow
K. severe, growing worse
L. relating to disease shifting through the body

133. _____ myelography	A.	painful nerves
134. _____ myoid	B.	growth of tissue with no purpose
135. _____ myoma	C.	inflammation of the bone
136. _____ neoplasm	D.	muscle tumor
137. _____ nephropexy	E.	inflammation of testicle
138. _____ nephrostomy	F.	muscle-like
139. _____ neuralgia	G.	study of the nerves
140. _____ neurology	H.	a picture of the spinal cord
141. _____ oophorectomy	I.	surgery on testicle
142. _____ orchidotomy	J.	operation to make a permanent opening in the kidney
143. _____ orchitis	K.	removal of ovary
144. _____ osteitis	L.	operation to fasten kidney in place

145. _____ ovary	A.	puncture of organs alongside cavity to release fluid
146. _____ paracentesis	B.	tumor on a stem
147. _____ pelvic	C.	tissue around anus
148. _____ pelvis	D.	inflammation of lining inside the abdomen
149. _____ perianal	E.	basin-shaped bones of lower trunk
150. _____ peripheral	F.	sudden collapse of lung
151. _____ peritonitis	G.	related to the outside of the body
152. _____ pneumonectomy	H.	inflammation of the lung
153. _____ pneumonia	I.	sex gland producing egg
154. _____ pneumonitis	J.	removal of lung
155. _____ pneumothorax	K.	relating to pelvis
156. _____ polyp	L.	congestion of lung

157. _____ proctoscopy	A.	gland surrounding bladder
158. _____ prognosis	B.	drop in blood pressure
159. _____ prostate	C.	instrumental exam of rectum
160. _____ prostatectomy	D.	protrusion of rectum
161. _____ proximal	E.	drooping of an organ
162. _____ ptosis	F.	free of all living germs
163. _____ radical resection	G.	part of limb nearest trunk
164. _____ rectocele	H.	containing pus-producing germs
165. _____ rectum	I.	removal of prostate
166. _____ septic	J.	surgical removal of organ and surrounding parts
167. _____ shock	K.	forecast of condition
168. _____ sterile	L.	last part of the large intestine

169. _____ stomach	A.	group of symptoms occurring together
170. _____ stroke	B.	relating to the entire body
171. _____ suture	C.	stretchy organ for collection of swallowed food
172. _____ symptom	D.	inflammation of the tendon
173. _____ syncope	E.	sign of disease
174. _____ syndrome	F.	puncture thorax to release air
175. _____ systemic	G.	fainting
176. _____ tachycardia	H.	fast heartbeat
177. _____ tenontitis	I.	stitch to hold wound closed
178. _____ testicle	J.	relating to the thorax
179. _____ thoracentesis	K.	bursting of blood vessel in brain
180. _____ thoracic	L.	male sex gland

181. ____ thoracotomy
182. ____ thorax
183. ____ thrombus
184. ____ thyroid
185. ____ thyroidectomy
186. ____ trachea
187. ____ tracheal endoscope
188. ____ tracheoscopy
189. ____ tracheotomy
190. ____ trauma
191. ____ tumor
192. ____ unsterile

A. not free of all living germs
B. bony cage of chest
C. instrument to look inside trachea
D. removal of thyroid
E. sudden drop in blood pressure
F. gland near upper part of trachea
G. growth of tissue with no purpose
H. cut thorax
I. cutting operation on trachea
J. blood clot
K. tube from mouth to lungs
L. examination of trachea with special instrument

193. ____ ureter
194. ____ ureterotomy
195. ____ urethra
196. ____ urethritis
197. ____ uterus
198. ____ vagina
199. ____ vaginitis
200. ____ vasospasm
201. ____ ventral
202. ____ vertigo

A. vessel cramp
B. inflammation of urethra
C. female organ of sexual intercourse
D. cutting operation of ureter
E. dizziness
F. tube carrying urine outside body
G. inflammation of vagina
H. pear-shaped organ called womb
I. front surface of the body
J. tube from kidney to bladder

Instructions
True/False & Fill-in-the-blanks

The preceding exercises were a listing of the words or word parts with a list of possible answers from which you were to select the correct one. The True/False and Fill-in-the Blank Exercises are somewhat different in that it is assumed—to varying degrees—that you have memorized a word's definition and can recite it on command. Such retention is the obvious aim of this course, but the best way to achieve this ability is to first learn to recognize the various components which make up each word.

In doing the following two exercises, study the key words (those which are all capitalized) before answering; try to remember the word/picture associations which correspond to each word or word part. In many cases you may be able to find the correct answer even though the entire word is not immediately familiar to you.

TRUE/FALSE

There are fifty true/false questions. Read each one carefully; then enter either the word ''true'' or ''false'' in the blank provided to the left of each question. For example:

False 1. Grass grows on trees.

True 2. Red is a color.

True 3. Ice is frozen water.

False 4. Most people live to be 200 years old.

Answers to the fifty true/false questions are found on page 154. Place an X next to all incorrect answers, and again refer to the word/picture associations and study those words you did not understand.

FILL-IN-THE-BLANK

There are sixty-five fill-in-the-blank questions, each one requiring that you write in at least one word which will correctly complete that sentence. You will note that at the end of each sentence there is a number (in some cases there are two numbers). This number (or numbers) tells you how many letters there are in the word or words you are to write in the blank. For example:

1. Ice is frozen *water* . (5)

2. Leaves grow on *trees* and are usually *green* in color.   (5;5)

Answers to these questions are given on page 155. Place an X next to all incorrect answers. Study the correct answer, again referring to the word/picture associations.

True/False Exercises

_______ 1. When two parts are said to ADHERE, it means that they stick together.

_______ 2. A CONCUSSION refers to injury to the back.

_______ 3. NEUROLOGY is the science dealing with the nerves.

_______ 4. HEMORRHAGE is the bursting forth of blood.

_______ 5. The URETER is the tube that runs from the kidney to the bladder.

_______ 6. A CORONARY THROMBOSIS is a heart attack due to a clot in the aorta.

_______ 7. MALAISE refers to a definite feeling of illness.

_______ 8. The COLON is the large intestine.

_______ 9. EDEMA is the condition of having fluid in the tissue.

_______ 10. When a condition is said to be ACQUIRED, it means that the person was born that way.

_______ 11. A THROMBUS is a blood clot.

_______ 12. EPISTAXIS is a headache due to anoxia.

_______ 13. The PROSTATE is the gland which surrounds the liver.

_______ 14. When something is ASEPTIC, it contains lots of germs.

_______ 15. The CEPHALUS is the whole head.

_______ 16. When a condition is said to be CONGENITAL, it means that it existed at birth.

_______ 17. A CHOLECYSTECTOMY is the removal of the kidney.

_______ 18. A PROCTOSCOPY is an instrumental examination of the rectum.

_______ 19. DISTAL refers to the part of the body closest to the trunk.

_______ 20. A BENIGN tumor is one that is not MALIGNANT.

_______ 21. The VAGINA is the female organ of sexual intercourse.

_______ 22. The PELVIS is the group of basin-shaped bones located in the chest.

_______ 23. An ANGIOSPASM is a cramp of the blood vessels.

_______ 24. CALCULUS is the white matter found in the teeth and bones.

_______ 25. The ESOPHAGUS is the tube connecting the mouth to the stomach.

_______ 26. A MYOMA is a tumor of the brain.

_______ 27. The BRONCHI are the windpipes which enter the stomach.

_______ 28. When something is STERILE, it is free of all living germs.

_______ 29. HYPERTROPHY refers to the degeneration of a body part.

_______ 30. ABDOMINOCENTESIS is the puncturing of the stomach to let out air.

_______ 31. MALIGNANT, a term usually associated with cancer, means "severe and growing worse."

_______ 32. A TUMOR is a growth of tissue with no functional purpose.

_______ 33. GASTROENTERITIS is the inflammation of the stomach and intestines.

_______ 34. In medical terms, an AIRWAY is what doctors take to get from one convention to another.

__________ 35. When something is SEPTIC, it contains pus-producing germs.

__________ 36. MENOPAUSE refers to a decrease in the flow of the monthly menses.

__________ 37. ENCEPHALOGRAPHY is an operation on the brain.

__________ 38. A SYMPTOM is a sign of recovery.

__________ 39. CEREBRUM refers to the whole brain.

__________ 40. HYSTEROTOMY is an operation involving the cutting of the UTERUS.

__________ 41. A LESION is the area of diseased tissue.

__________ 42. The THYROID is the gland near the upper part of the skull.

__________ 43. DORSAL refers to the back side of the body.

__________ 44. A SUTURE is a stitch used to hold a wound closed.

__________ 45. ILEUM is the technical term for the heart.

__________ 46. An ANGIOSPASM is a cramp in the blood vessels.

__________ 47. A TRACHEOTOMY is an examination of the TRACHEA with a special instrument.

__________ 48. When something is SYSTEMIC, it refers to the entire body.

__________ 49. INTERNAL refers to the inside of the body.

__________ 50. A SYNDROME is a group of SYMPTOMS that occur separately.

Fill-in-the-blanks

1. A FRACTURE is a ________________ in the bone.   (5)

2. PERITONITIS is the inflammation of the lining inside the ________________.   (7)

3. VENTRAL refers to the ________________ surface of the body.   (5)

4. The INTESTINE is the lower ________________ tract.   (9)

5. The ABDOMEN is the cavity which contains the ________________.   (7)

6. The suffix which means "to cut to make a permanent opening" is ________________.   (5)

7. ENTERITIS is an ________________ of the intestine.   (12)

8. When a condition is CHRONIC, it recurs ________________.   (10)

9. The prefix meaning "skin" is ________________.   (5)

10. An ACUTE condition is one that is of ________________ course and ________________ duration.   (5;5)

11. The THORAX is the bony cage of the ________________.   (5)

12. APOPLEXY refers to paralysis and fainting due to ________________.   (6)

13. MYELOGRAPHY is a picture of the ________________.   (6;4)

14. The BLADDER is a sac-like structure which collects ________________.   (5)

15. Something is said to be ________________ when it contains pus-producing germs.   (5)

16. A STROKE involves the bursting of blood vessels in the ________________.   (5)

17. The prefix meaning "over" or "excessive" is ________________.   (5)

18. The UTERUS is the pear-shaped organ commonly called the ________________.   (4)

19. When a person suffers from ARTHRITIS, he or she has ________________ of the ________________.   (12;6)

20. FIBRILLATION is a fast ________________.   (9)

21. CEREBRAL means "relating to the ________________."   (5)

22. A tear in the skin is called a ________________.   (10)

23. SHOCK relates to a drop in ________________.   (5;8)

24. The identification of a condition is called the ________________.   (9)

25. NEURALGIA is the condition of painful ________________.   (6)

26. The prefix which means "HEART" is ________________.   (5)

27. EXCISION is removal by ________________.   (7;3)

28. When something is not free of all living germs, it is said to be ________________.   (9)

29. The GALL BLADDER is the sac that stores ________________.   (4)

30. The TRACHEA is the tube running from the ________________ to the ________________.   (5;5)

31. CYSTOCELE refers to the protrusion of the ________________.   (7)

32. A ________________ is a forecast of the future condition of a patient in relation to recovery.   (9)

33. METASTATIC means "relating to disease _________________ through the body." (8)

34. CAUTERIZATION refers to the destruction of tissue by _______________. (7)

35. HEMATOLOGY is the science dealing with the study of the _______________. (5)

36. The _______________ is the organ in which food is collected after being swallowed. (7)

37. The suffix meaning "picture of" is _______________. (6)

38. CYANOSIS is the "_______________ appearance of the _______________ due to ANOXIA." (4;4)

39. OSTEITIS is an inflammation of the _______________. (4)

40. A CARDIAC ARREST is a stoppage of the _______________. (5)

41. DYSPNEA refers to the difficulty in _______________ due to a blocked AIRWAY. (9)

42. The suffix which means "to remove surgically" is _______________. (6)

43. The _______________ is the organ that produces bile. (5)

44. When something is free of all living germs, it is said to be _______________. (7)

45. The protrusion of an organ through a wall or cavity is called a _______________. (6)

46. The two suffixes which mean "related to" are _______________ and _______________. (2;2)

47. A COMA is a state of deep _______________. (15)

48. The _______________ is the sex gland which produces the egg. (5)

49. DYSURIA refers to painful _______________. (9)

50. ANOREXIA refers to a loss of _______________. (8)

51. MENINGITIS is the _______________ of the brain covering. (12)

52. The muscular organ, located between the LUNGS, which pumps blood to the entire body is the _______________. (5)

53. The suffix that means "resembling" is _______________. (3)

54. A CONTUSION is a _______________. (6)

55. PNEUMONIA is an inflammation of the _______________. (5)

56. HEPATITIS is an inflammation of the _______________. (5)

57. CONVULSION refers to _______________ body movements. (9)

58. The suffix which means "to puncture, to let out air or fluid" is _______________. (8)

59. _______________ means occurring outside the body, or in an abnormal place; _______________ means occurring in the normal place. (7;7)

60. The _______________ is the organ that manufactures urine. (6)

61. CRANIAL means relating to the _______________. (5)

62. When something is free of all pus-producing germs, it is said to be _______________. (5)

63. The URETHRA is the tube that carries _______________ outside the body. (5)

64. A bladder-like sac containing fluid is called a _______________. (4)

65. The _______________ is an organ for which there is little or no biological use; located off the large intestine, on the right side of the body. (8)

Re-test Instructions

You have now completed the various exercises designed to increase your understanding of those words which are a part of your daily profession. In addition you have studied the word/picture associations designed to give you some memory key on which to base your retention of the word and its definition.

The first exercise you took included all 202 Index words in the form of multiple choice questions. This "pre-test" gave you some idea of the number of words you had to learn. Now that you have completed the subsequent exercises, you will take a "re-test." It is exactly the same exercise as the "pre-test," and you should follow all the same directions.

The answer sheet for this exercise follows on page 133. Turn back to page 3 and again read each word. Choose the best definition and place the number on your answer sheet. Try to remember the word/picture associations.

When you have finished, turn to page 151 and check your answers. Then record the number you answered correctly in the space provided.

Re-test Answer Sheet

NAME_______________________

1. ___	27. ___	53. ___	79. ___	105. ___	131. ___	157. ___	180. ___
2. ___	28. ___	54. ___	80. ___	106. ___	132. ___	158. ___	181. ___
3. ___	29. ___	55. ___	81. ___	107. ___	133. ___	159. ___	182. ___
4. ___	30. ___	56. ___	82. ___	108. ___	134. ___	160. ___	183. ___
5. ___	31. ___	57. ___	83. ___	109. ___	135. ___	161. ___	184. ___
6. ___	32. ___	58. ___	84. ___	110. ___	136. ___	162. ___	185. ___
7. ___	33. ___	59. ___	85. ___	111. ___	137. ___	163. ___	186. ___
8. ___	34. ___	60. ___	86. ___	112. ___	138. ___	164. ___	187. ___
9. ___	35. ___	61. ___	87. ___	113. ___	139. ___	165. ___	188. ___
10. ___	36. ___	62. ___	88. ___	114. ___	140. ___	166. ___	189. ___
11. ___	37. ___	63. ___	89. ___	115. ___	141. ___	167. ___	190. ___
12. ___	38. ___	64. ___	90. ___	116. ___	142. ___	168. ___	191. ___
13. ___	39. ___	65. ___	91. ___	117. ___	143. ___	169. ___	192. ___
14. ___	40. ___	66. ___	92. ___	118. ___	144. ___	170. ___	193. ___
15. ___	41. ___	67. ___	93. ___	119. ___	145. ___	171. ___	194. ___
16. ___	42. ___	68. ___	94. ___	120. ___	146. ___	172. ___	195. ___
17. ___	43. ___	69. ___	95. ___	121. ___	147. ___	173. ___	196. ___
18. ___	44. ___	70. ___	96. ___	122. ___	148. ___	174. ___	197. ___
19. ___	45. ___	71. ___	97. ___	123. ___	149. ___	175. ___	198. ___
20. ___	46. ___	72. ___	98. ___	124. ___	150. ___	176. ___	199. ___
21. ___	47. ___	73. ___	99. ___	125. ___	151. ___	177. ___	200. ___
22. ___	48. ___	74. ___	100. ___	126. ___	152. ___	178. ___	201. ___
23. ___	49. ___	75. ___	101. ___	127. ___	153. ___	179. ___	202. ___
24. ___	50. ___	76. ___	102. ___	128. ___	154. ___		
25. ___	51. ___	77. ___	103. ___	129. ___	155. ___	SCORE _______	
26. ___	52. ___	78. ___	104. ___	130. ___	156. ___		

CROSSWORD
PUZZLES

Instructions

The following crossword puzzles are designed to be completed in conjunction with the other exercises. Your instructor will tell you when you should work these puzzles, or you may refer to the Self-Instruction Program Sheet at the back of this book.

The first three puzzles consist solely of suffixes and prefixes. You simply read the definition given and write the word, letter by letter, in the blocks, either across or down from the corresponding number.

Follow this same procedure for the three whole-word puzzles. In these last three puzzles, part of many words have already been filled in. These words are difficult, so if you are unable to remember the word or its correct spelling you may refer to the word/picture association section and look for the answer. The solutions to these puzzles are found on pages 156 through 161. Check your answers; always study the word/picture associations for those words you were not able to remember.

Suffix Puzzle

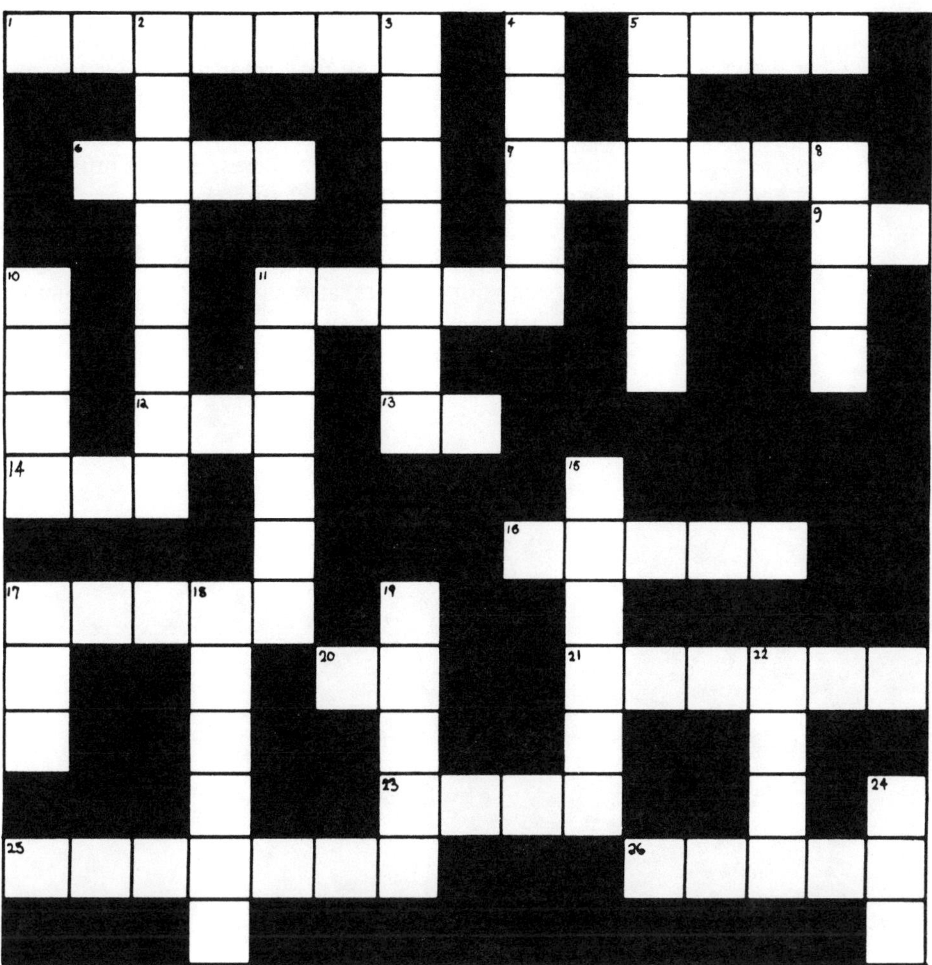

Across

1. Tissue or organ
5. Cut; make a permanent opening
6. Breath
7. Knowledge of condition
9. Condition of
11. Oxygen
12. Character of
13. Related to
14. Process; condition
16. Sticking out of an organ
17. Knowledge of
20. Related to
21. Cessation; stoppage
23. To fasten surgically
25. Burst forth
26. Contraction of; cramp

Down

2. To puncture; to let out air or fluid
3. Appetite
4. Painful
5. Growth
8. Condition of being
10. Inflammation of
11. Normal
15. Remove surgically
17. Resemble
18. Picture of
19. Instrument used to examine or look at; to examine
22. Urination
24. Tumor

Prefix Puzzle I

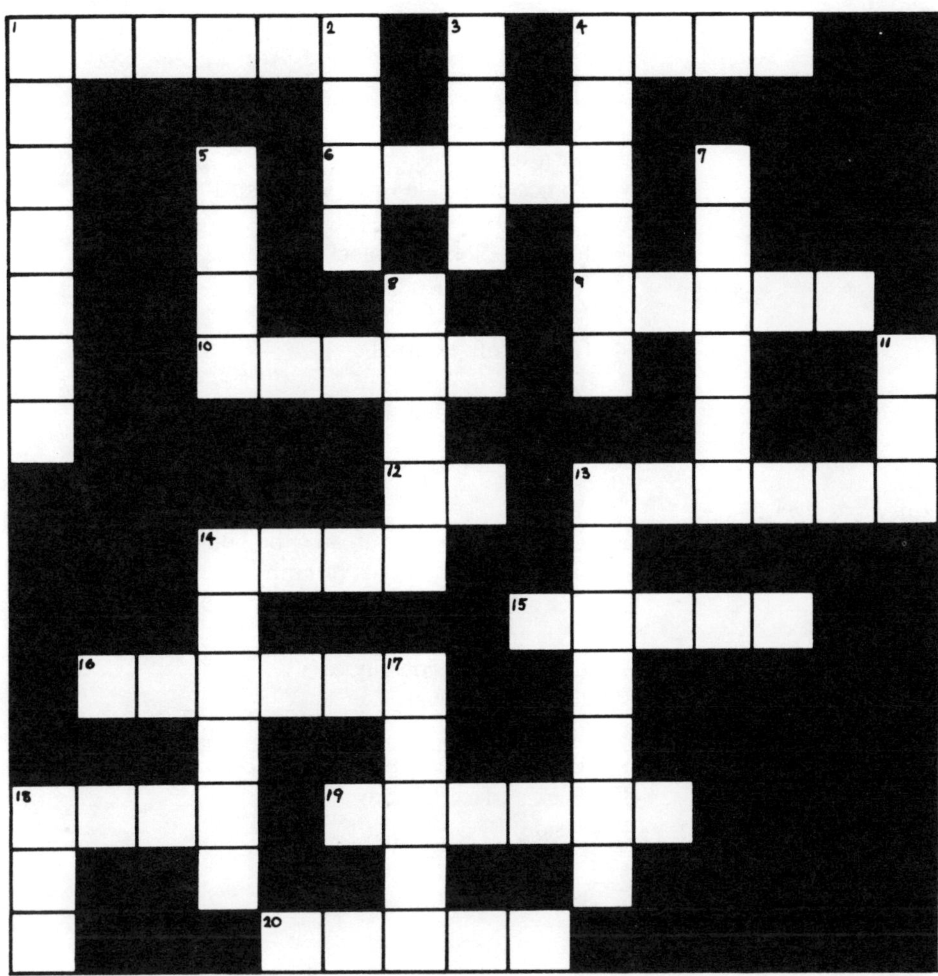

Across

1. Tear or cut in skin
4. Fibrous tissue
6. Water
9. Intestine
10. Abdomen
12. Slow down; decrease
13. Jarring injury to the brain
14. Around
15. Bruise
16. Part of limb nearest trunk
18. Part of limb furthest away from trunk
19. Kidney
20. Gall

Down

1. Voice box
2. Abnormal sticking together
3. Inside
4. Rapid examination of tissue
5. Bile
7. Away from body surface
8. Heart
11. Difficulty; painful
13. Cartilage
14. Rectum
17. Spinal cord
18. Identification

Prefix Puzzle II

Across

1. Liver
3. Existing at birth
6. Remove by cutting out
8. Vessel
9. Nerves
10. Slow
11. Occurring in a normal place
12. Muscle
13. Ovary
15. Bone
17. Long duration; recurring frequently
18. Forecast
20. Lung
21. Join two parts to make a new passageway
23. Drooping of an organ
25. Breathing
27. Stomach
28. Malignant
29. Spit blood from lungs
33. Painful menses
36. None, not
37. Gland; glandular tissue
39. Skin
41. Lining inside of abdomen
42. Ballooning out of blood vessel at weak point

Down

1. Uterus
2. Joints
3. Burn tissue
4. To occur outside or in an unusual place
5. Fast
6. Floating bloodclot blocking the vessel
7. Blue appearance of skin
12. Monthly flow
14. Outside of; external
16. Tendon
19. Heart attack due to blocked coronary vessel
22. Blood vessel
24. Testicle
25. Vessel
26. Limited to specific area of the body
28. Irregular movements of limbs
30. Disease shifting from one part of the body to another
31. Organs alongside any cavity
32. Over; excessively
34. Inside
35. Blood
38. Back surface of body
40. Inside

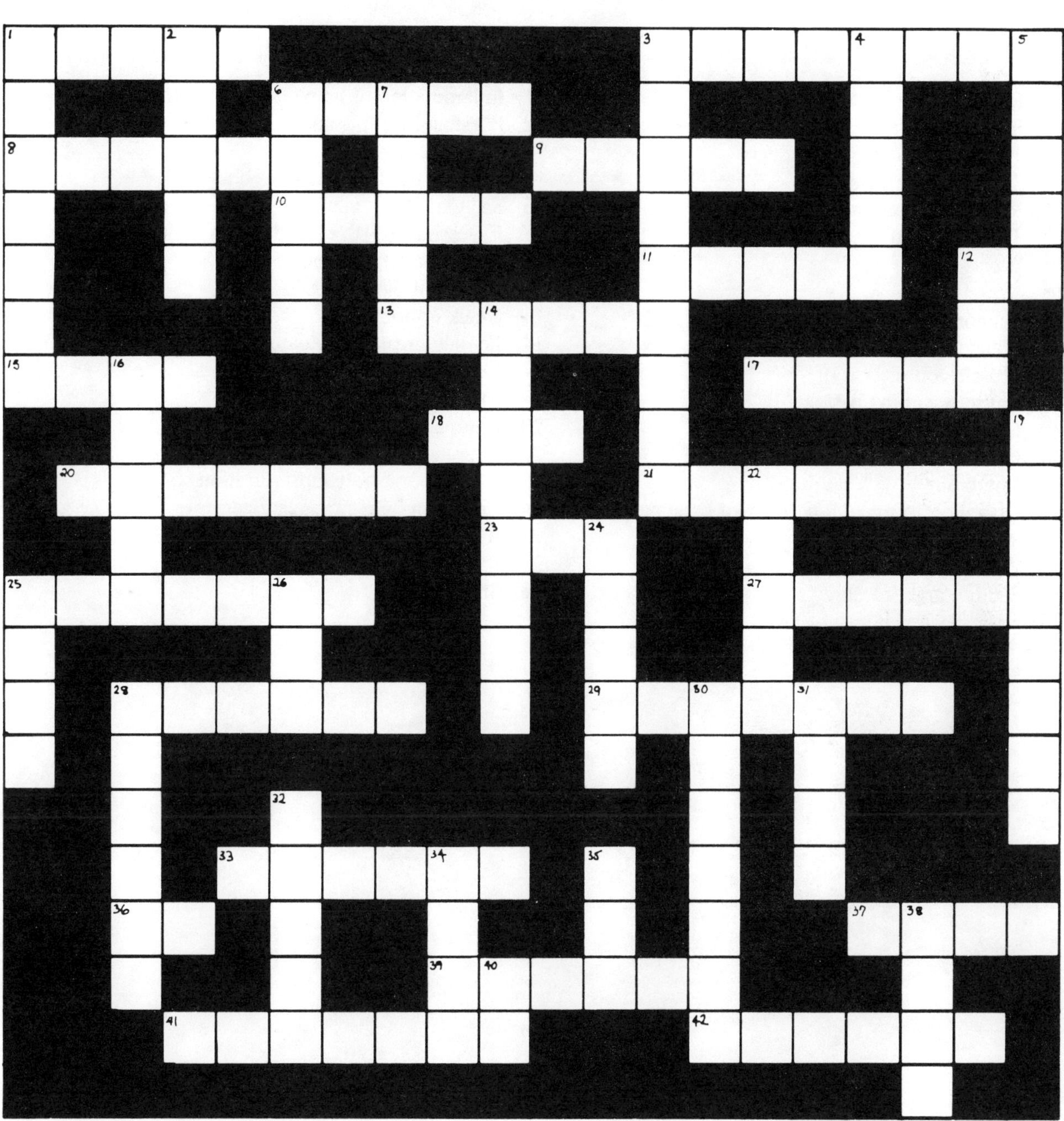

Whole Word Puzzle I

<table>
<tr><td valign="top" width="50%">

Across

1. Related to the outside of the body
4. Removal of tissue for microscopic examination
6. Tube from kidney to bladder
8. Surgery on testicle
11. Rapid examination of tissue
12. Tissue around anus
13. Bruise
15. Vessel cramp
16. Balloon-like structures in chest
18. Malignant tumor
22. Muscle contraction of voice box
26. Entire breathing passage
29. Cutting operation of trachea
30. Cut thorax
31. The brain
32. Operation to make a permanent opening in the kidney
33. Fibrous tumor
34. Sac off large intestine
35. Basin-shaped bones of lower trunk

</td><td valign="top" width="50%">

Down

1. Inflammation of lining inside abdomen
2. Bursting forth of blood
3. Glandular tissue tumor
4. To look inside bronchi
5. Sac that stores bile
7. Excessive growth of body parts
9. Inflammation of urethra
10. Picture of blood vessels
11. Crack in bone
14. Female organ of sexual intercourse
17. Relating to the brain
19. Cutting operation of ureter
20. Last part of the large intestine
21. Operation to fasten kidney in place
23. Rapid course and short duration
24. Containing pus-producing germs
25. Relating to abdomen
27. Painful urination
28. Small intestine

</td></tr>
</table>

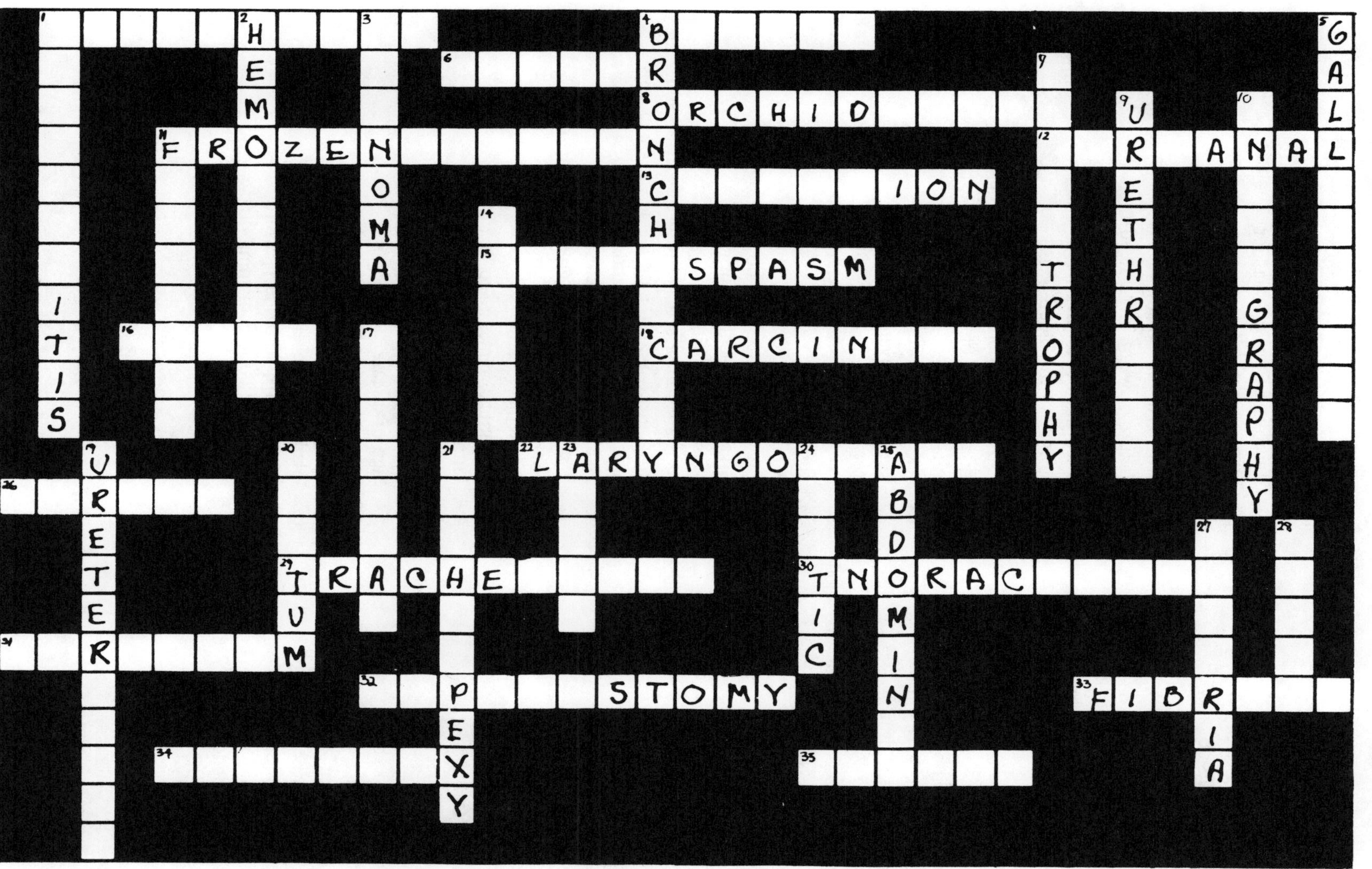

Whole Word Puzzle II

Across

1. Bursting of brain blood vessel
6. Picture showing inside of head
10. Tube carrying urine outside body
14. Bloodclot
15. Fast heartbeat
16. Blue appearance of skin due to anoxia
17. Tube from mouth to stomach
19. Bursting of blood vessel in the brain
21. Tear in skin
22. Large intestine
25. Containing pus-producing germs
26. Bony cage of chest
28. Instrument examination of the bladder
29. Reaction occurring after injection of drug due to allergy to the drug
32. Back surface of body
33. Stretchy organ for collection of swallowed food
37. Painful flow of monthly menses
38. Drop in blood pressure
39. Bleeding from lungs
44. Fainting
46. Removal of thyroid
48. To cut into the abdomen
50. Slow heartbeat electrically
51. Fluid in abdominal cavity
52. Relating to the head
53. Existing at birth
56. Overbreathing
58. Cutting the skull
60. Skin tumor
62. Tube from mouth to lungs
65. Injury to the brain
66. Removal of prostate
67. Ballooning out of blood vessel
68. Removal of lung
69. Sex gland producing egg
70. Puncture thorax to release air
71. Puncture of organs alongside cavity to release fluid
72. Heart attack due to bloodclot in coronary vessels

Down

1. Removal of the gall bladder
2. Surgical removal of an organ and surrounding parts
3. Gland-like
4. Protrusion of rectum
5. Picture of water inside head
6. Nosebleed
7. Deep unconsciousness
8. Science of the blood
9. Loss of appetite
11. Temporary stoppage of breathing
12. Inflammation of cartilage
13. Inflammation of stomach and intestine
18. Science of nerves
20. Removal of ovary
22. Recurring frequently
23. Part of limb furthest from trunk
24. The head
27. A picture of the spinal cord
30. Growth of tissue with no purpose
31. Organ manufacturing urine
34. Muscle-like
35. Examination of bronchi with a special instrument
36. Instrument used to look inside the esophagus
40. Inflammation of the tendon
41. Stitch to hold wound closed
42. Examination of esophagus with instrument
43. Slow heartbeat
45. The skull
47. Abdominal puncture to let out air
49. Tumor on a stem
54. Inflammation of joints
55. Gland surrounding bladder
57. Sign of disease
59. Inflammation of bone
61. Shortage of oxygen
62. Gland near upper part of trachea
63. Sudden drop in blood pressure
64. Bladder-like sac containing fluid

RADICAL
RECT
ENCEPHAL
TACHY
XIA
ENTER
SIS
ENCEPHAL
ECTOMY
OSCOPY
TOL
SHOC K
OGY
IC
ESOPHAGEAL
BRONCHI
THYROID
ATION
LAPAR
ABDOMINO
IC CON
ATION
OTOMY
TOMA
PROSTAT
ECTOMY
THORA
CENTESIS
CORONARY

Whole Word Puzzle III

Across

2. Instrument to look inside trachea
7. Stoppage of the heart
11. Sudden collapse of lung
13. Drooping of an organ
14. Relating to the entire body
16. The part of the body away from the surface
17. Occurring outside the body
20. Inflammation of the vagina
21. Congestion of the lung
22. Vessel cramp
23. Relating to the pelvis
25. Fast heartbeat
29. Cutting to make permanent opening
   in small intestine
30. Vary from normal
33. Excessive menstrual flow
36. Brain covering
37. Free of all living germs
41. Vague feeling of illness
42. Organ producing bile
44. Growth of tissue with no purpose
45. Sickness
46. Protrusion of the bladder
50. Inflammation of testicle
51. Occurring in normal place
54. Relating to inside of trachea
56. Right and left windpipes which enter lungs
58. Specific area of body
60. Part of limb nearest trunk
61. Free of pus-producing germs
63. Cavity containing stomach
68. Dizziness
69. Stoppage of monthly menses flow
70. Free of pus-producing germs
73. A stone
75. Water hernia in testicle
76. The shifting of disease from one part of
   the body to another
77. Herniation of brain cover
78. Forecast of condition
79. Inflammation of the liver
80. Destroy tissue by burning
81. Not free of all living germs
82. Removal of appendix

Down

1. Paralysis and fainting due to stroke
3. Opening at end of digestive tract
4. Inflammation of intestine
5. Headache
6. Inflammation of the lung
7. Formation of gall stones
8. Join two parts together to make a new passageway
9. Blocking of vessel by traveling bloodclot
10. Examination of trachea with special instrument
12. Front surface of the body
15. Irregular body movements
18. Difficulty breathing due to blocked airway
19. Lower digestive tract
24. Fluid in the tissue
26. Painful joints
27. Resembling fibrous tissue
28. Resembling skin
31. Inflammation of brain covering
32. Mild and not recurring
34. Fastening of uterus in place
35. Wasting away of body parts
38. Area of diseased tissue
39. Male sex gland
40. Cutting of uterus
43. Painful stomach
44. Painful nerves
47. Group of symptoms occurring together
48. Developed after birth
49. The science of the heart
52. Instrumental exam of rectum
53. Convulsion before or after birth
55. Operation to make permanent hole in large intestine
56. Sac-like structure collecting urine
57. Relating to the skull
59. Identification of condition
62. Relating to the thorax
64. Muscle tumor
65. Make permanent opening in intestine
66. Relating to disease shifting through body
67. Severe, growing worse
71. Remove by cutting out
72. Muscular organ between lungs
73. Malignant tumor
74. Pear-shaped organ called womb
75. Protrusion of organ through wall or cavity

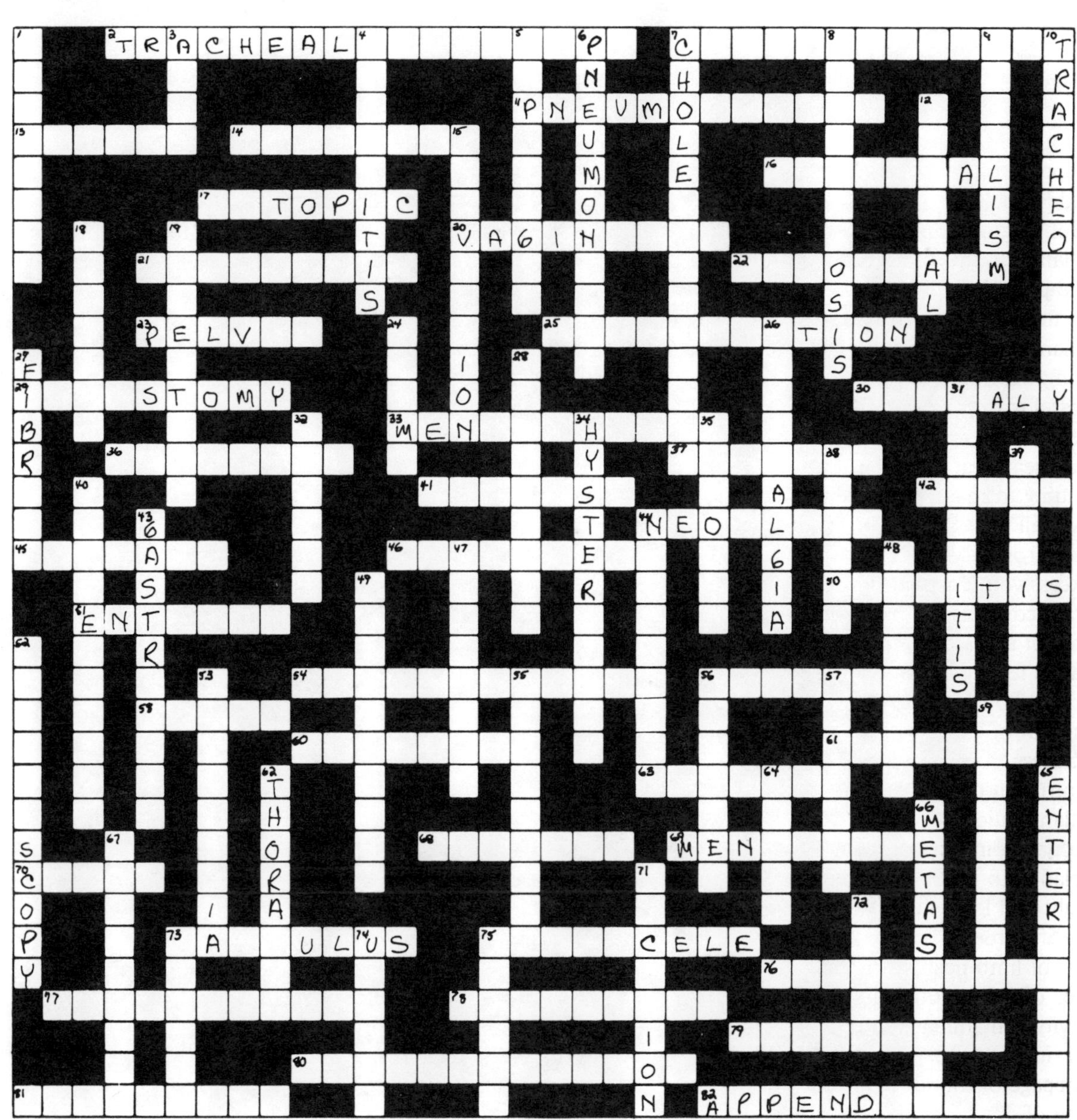

ANSWER SECTION

Pre-test/Re-test Answers

1. 3	27. 4	53. 1	79. 1	105. 1	131. 3	157. 2	180. 1
2. 3	28. 3	54. 1	80. 4	106. 4	132. 3	158. 4	181. 2
3. 4	29. 3	55. 3	81. 4	107. 3	133. 3	159. 4	182. 4
4. 1	30. 4	56. 4	82. 3	108. 2	134. 1	160. 1	183. 1
5. 2	31. 2	57. 2	83. 3	109. 3	135. 4	161. 2	184. 1
6. 3	32. 1	58. 2	84. 2	110. 3	136. 2	162. 4	185. 2
7. 2	33. 4	59. 3	85. 3	111. 2	137. 1	163. 4	186. 2
8. 1	34. 2	60. 3	86. 2	112. 1	138. 1	164. 1	187. 3
9. 4	35. 3	61. 2	87. 3	113. 3	139. 4	165. 2	188. 1
10. 1	36. 3	62. 2	88. 1	114. 1	140. 4	166. 3	189. 4
11. 3	37. 1	63. 3	89. 4	115. 2	141. 2	167. 4	190. 1
12. 4	38. 1	64. 1	90. 2	116. 1	142. 3	168. 2	191. 1
13. 2	39. 3	65. 4	91. 4	117. 3	143. 3	169. 3	192. 1
14. 4	40. 1	66. 1	92. 2	118. 4	144. 2	170. 4	193. 2
15. 4	41. 4	67. 4	93. 1	119. 1	145. 4	171. 2	194. 3
16. 3	42. 3	68. 2	94. 4	120. 3	146. 1	172. 4	195. 2
17. 3	43. 2	69. 3	95. 2	121. 3	147. 3	173. 2	196. 4
18. 2	44. 1	70. 2	96. 1	122. 1	148. 2	174. 3	197. 1
19. 2	45. 1	71. 4	97. 2	123. 1	149. 4	175. 1	198. 1
20. 4	46. 2	72. 2	98. 4	124. 2	150. 4	176. 4	199. 3
21. 2	47. 3	73. 1	99. 1	125. 1	151. 1	177. 1	200. 1
22. 3	48. 1	74. 3	100. 3	126. 4	152. 2	178. 4	201. 1
23. 3	49. 2	75. 3	101. 3	127. 4	153. 4	179. 2	202. 1
24. 1	50. 4	76. 2	102. 1	128. 1	154. 2		
25. 1	51. 2	77. 2	103. 2	129. 2	155. 4		
26. 2	52. 4	78. 4	104. 1	130. 4	156. 1		

Matching Answers

PREFIXES

1. C	37. F
2. G	38. I
3. J	39. D
4. F	40. J
5. H	41. L
6. A	42. A
7. L	43. G
8. I	44. E
9. D	45. B
10. K	46. K
11. B	47. H
12. E	48. C
13. C	49. F
14. H	50. D
15. G	51. H
16. A	52. L
17. E	53. K
18. K	54. E
19. I	55. A
20. J	56. J
21. B	57. G
22. L	58. C
23. F	59. I
24. D	60. B
25. J	61. G
26. B	62. D
27. L	63. F
28. E	64. C
29. I	65. K
30. A or D	66. B
31. A or D	67. M
32. K	68. L
33. G	69. E
34. F	70. J
35. H	71. H
36. C	72. I
	73. A

SUFFIXES

1. H or J
2. D
3. F
4. C
5. A
6. I
7. G
8. H or J
9. B
10. E
11. B
12. F
13. I
14. H
15. J
16. A
17. E
18. D
19. G
20. C
21. B
22. E
23. G
24. I
25. D
26. C
27. A
28. H
29. F

1. J	47. F	92. D	137. L	181. H
2. D	48. H	93. L	138. J	182. B
3. F		94. F	139. A	183. J
4. L	49. G	95. J	140. G	184. F
5. B	50. K	96. B	141. K	185. D
6. H	51. E		142. I	186. K
7. A	52. A	97. A	143. E	187. C
8. E	53. I	98. E	144. C	188. L
9. G	54. C	99. G		189. I
10. I	55. J	100. K	145. I	190. E
11. C	56. F	101. C	146. A	191. G
12. K	57. L	102. I	147. K	192. A
	58. B	103. D	148. E	
13. H	59. D	104. F	149. C	193. J
14. D	60. H	105. B	150. G	194. D
15. L		106. H	151. D	195. F
16. F	61. F	107. L	152. J	196. B
17. B	62. B	108. J	153. L	197. H
18. J	63. J		154. H	198. C
19. K	64. L	109. B	155. F	199. G
20. C	65. D	110. D	156. B	200. A
21. G	66. H	111. L		201. I
22. I	67. E	112. H	157. C	202. E
23. A	68. I	113. F	158. K	
24. E	69. K	114. J	159. A	
	70. A	115. I	160. I	
25. G	71. G	116. C	161. G	
26. E	72. C	117. G	162. E	
27. I		118. K	163. J	
28. C	73. B	119. A	164. D	
29. A	74. L	120. E	165. L	
30. K	75. D		166. H	
31. H	76. H	121. I	167. B	
32. J	77. J	122. C	168. F	
33. L	78. F	123. G		
34. D	79. I	124. A	169. C	
35. F	80. C	125. K	170. K	
36. B	81. K	126. E	171. I	
	82. G	127. H	172. E	
37. A	83. A	128. B	173. G	
38. K	84. E	129. D	174. A	
39. G		130. J	175. B	
40. I	85. E	131. F	176. H	
41. E	86. K	132. L	177. D	
42. C	87. I		178. L	
43. L	88. C	133. H	179. F	
44. D	89. A	134. F	180. J	
45. B	90. G	135. D		
46. J	91. H	136. B		

True/False Answers

1. True
2. False (It refers to injury to the brain.)
3. True
4. True
5. True
6. False (It is a heart attack due to a clot in the coronary vessels.)
7. False (It is a vague feeling of illness.)
8. True
9. True
10. False (It means developed after birth.)
11. True
12. False (It is a nosebleed.)
13. False (It surrounds the bladder.)
14. False (It is free of all pus-producing germs.)
15. True
16. True
17. False (It is the removal of the gall bladder.)
18. True
19. False (It refers to the part furthest from the trunk.)
20. True
21. True
22. False (They are located in the lower trunk.)
23. True
24. False (It is a stone.)
25. True
26. False (It is a muscle cramp.)
27. False (They enter the lungs.)
28. True
29. False (It refers to the excessive growth of a body part.)
30. True
31. True
32. True
33. True
34. False (It is the entire breathing passage.)
35. True
36. False (It refers to the stoppage of menses.)
37. False (It is a picture of the inside of the head.)
38. False (It is a sign of disease.)
39. True
40. True
41. True
42. False (It is the gland near the upper part of the trachea.)
43. True
44. True
45. False (It is the small intestine.)
46. True
47. False (It is an operation on the trachea.)
48. True
49. True
50. False (It is a group of symptoms occurring together.)

Fill-in-the-blanks Answers

1. crack
2. ABDOMEN
3. front
4. digestive
5. STOMACH
6. tomy (or otomy or stomy)
7. inflammation
8. frequently
9. derma
10. rapid; short
11. chest
12. STROKE
13. spinal cord
14. urine
15. DIRTY
16. brain
17. hyper
18. womb
19. inflammation; joints
20. heartbeat
21. brain
22. LACERATION
23. blood pressure
24. DIAGNOSIS
25. nerves
26. cardi
27. cutting out
28. UNSTERILE
29. bile
30. mouth; lungs
31. BLADDER
32. PROGNOSIS
33. shifting
34. burning
35. blood
36. STOMACH
37. graphy
38. blue; skin
39. bone
40. HEART
41. breathing
42. ectomy
43. LIVER
44. STERILE
45. HERNIA
46. al; ic
47. unconsciousness
48. OVARY
49. urination
50. appetite
51. inflammation
52. HEART

53. oid
54. bruise
55. LUNGS
56. LIVER
57. irregular
58. centesis
59. ECTOPIC; ENTOPIC
60. KIDNEY
61. skull
62. CLEAN
63. urine
64. CYST
65. APPENDIX

Suffix Puzzle Solution

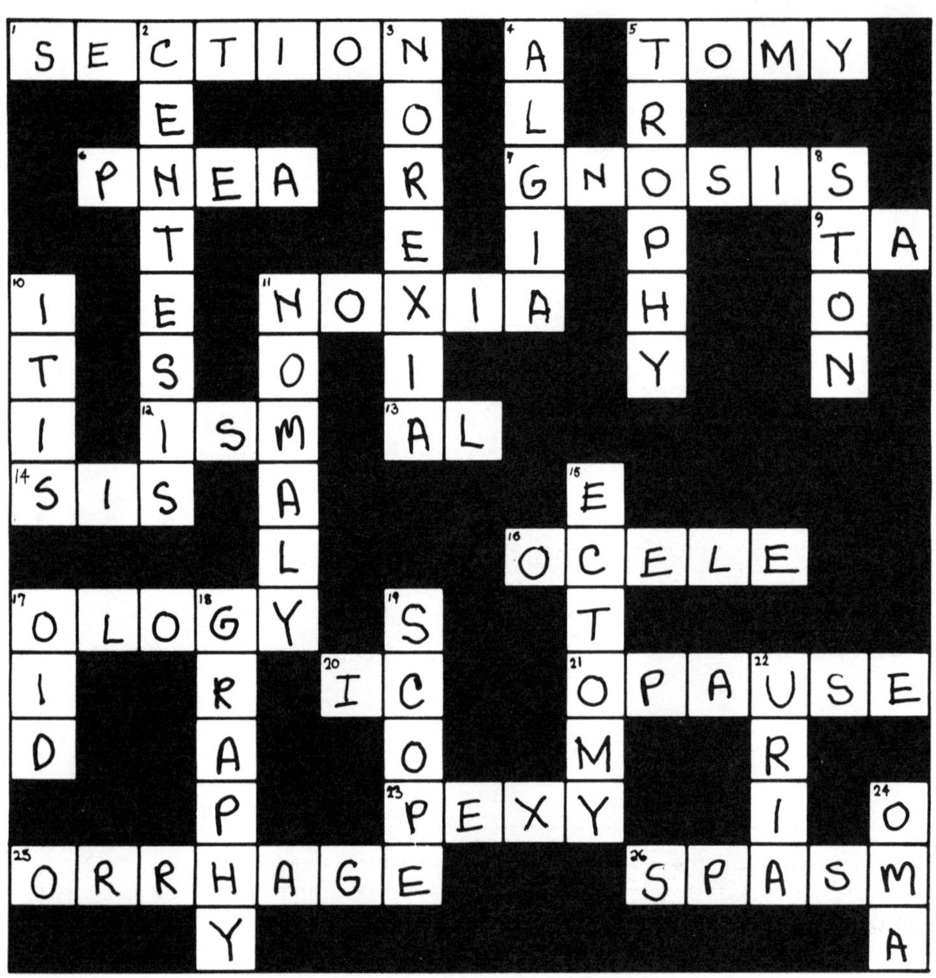

Prefix Puzzle I Solution

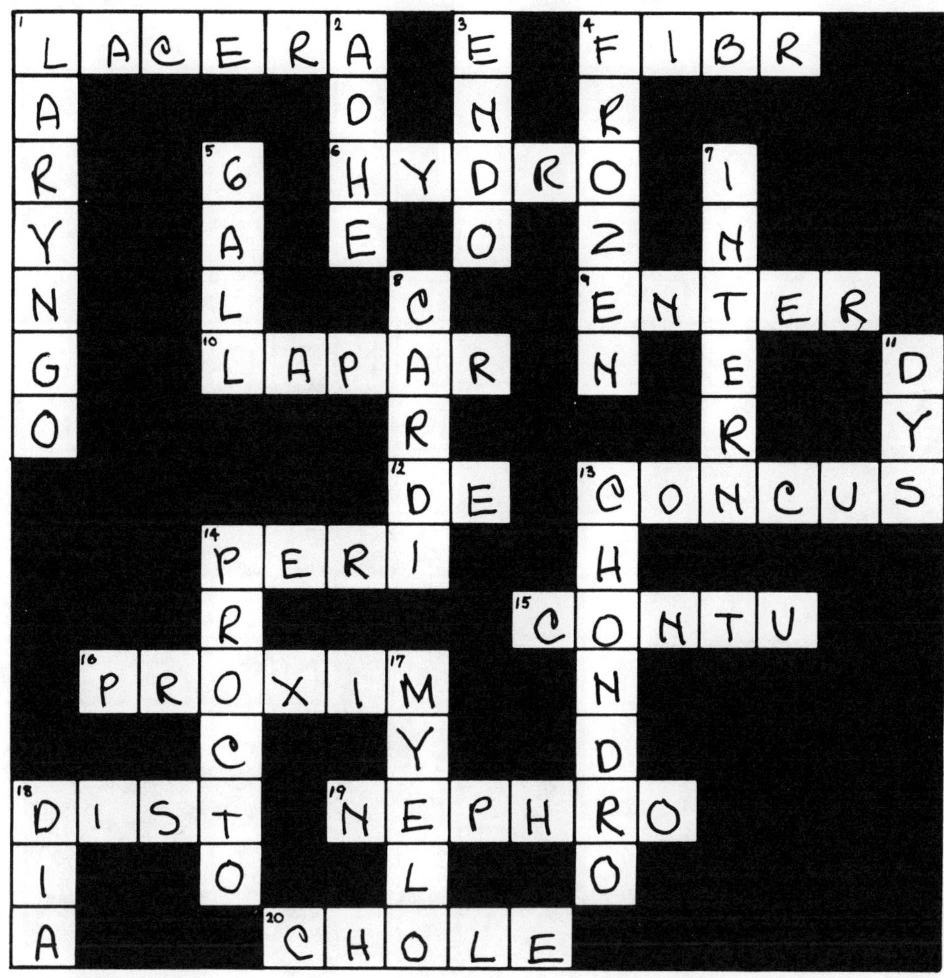

Prefix Puzzle II Solution

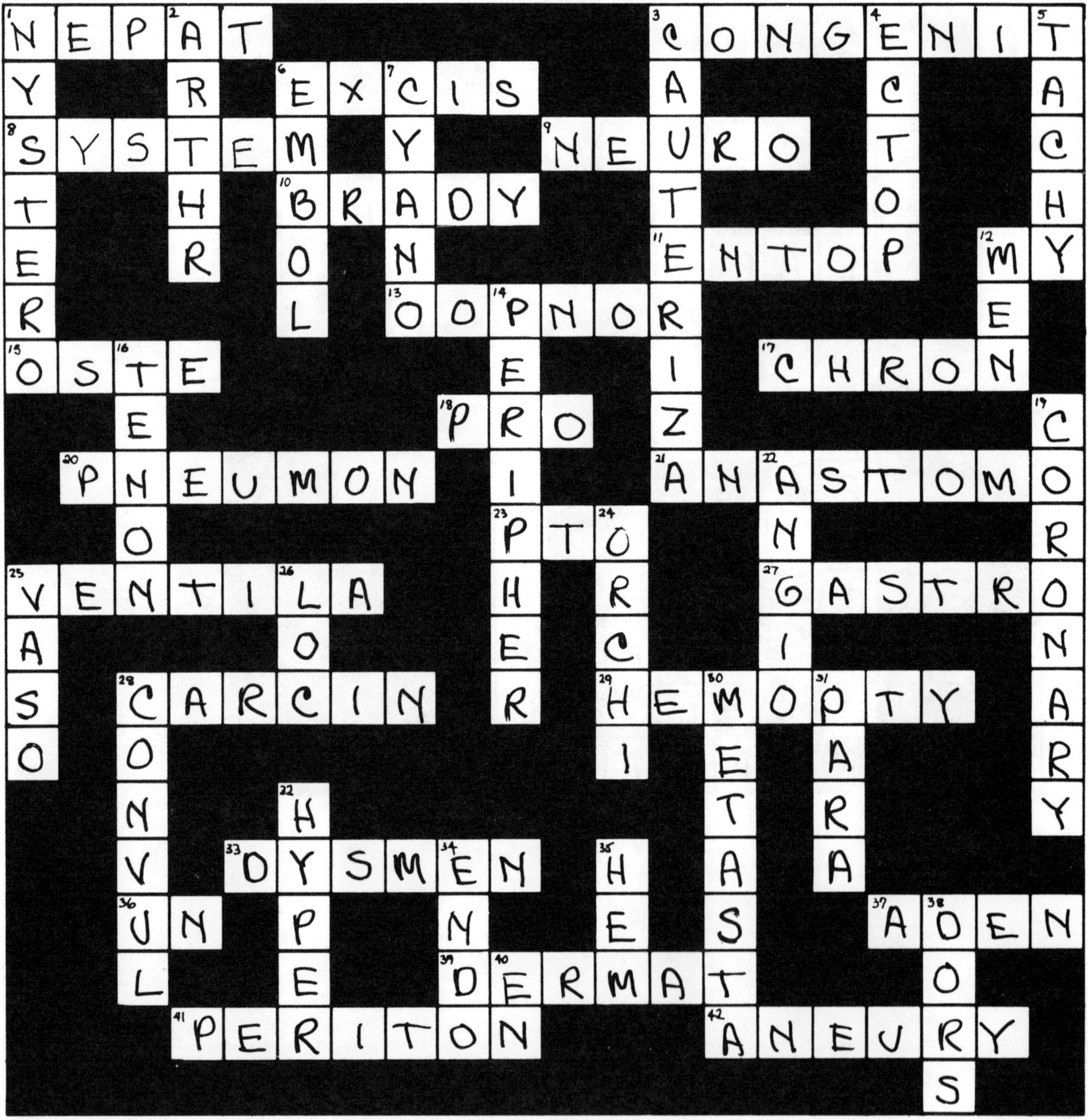

Whole Word Puzzle I Solution

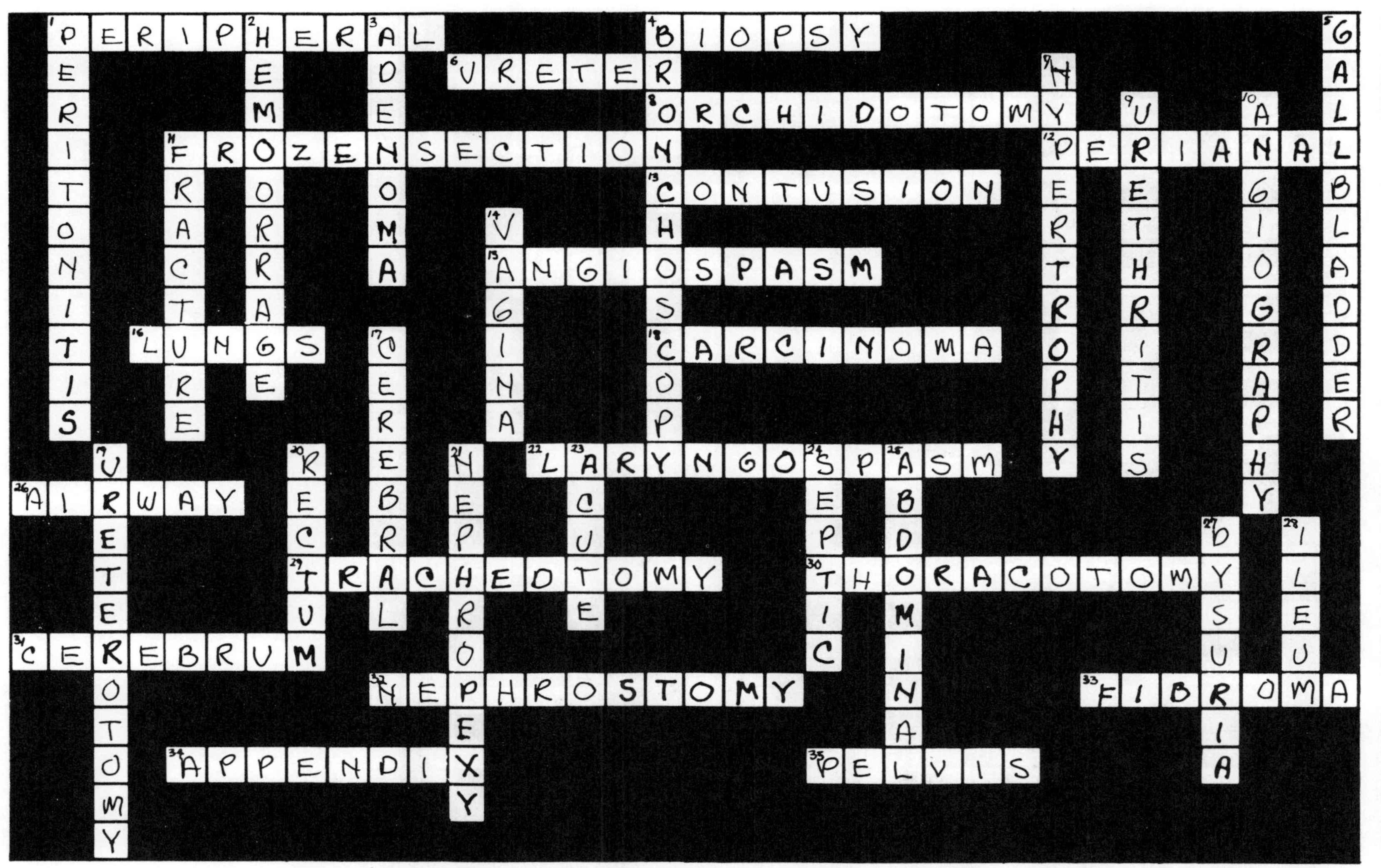

Whole Word Puzzle II Solution

Whole Words Puzzle III Solution

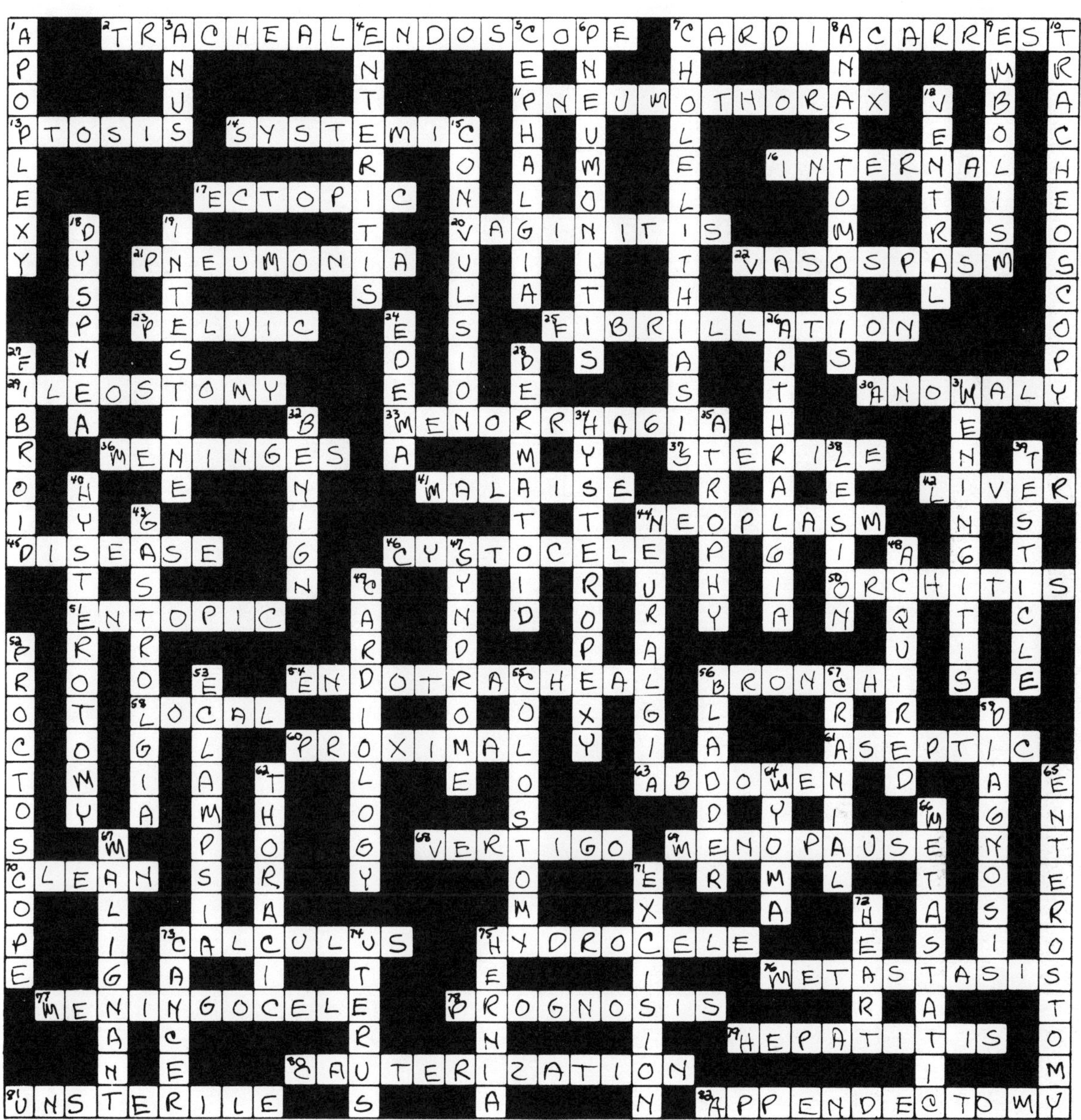

Program Score Sheet

PRE-TEST EXERCISE
Out of 202 terms, I correctly identified __173__.

PREFIX MATCHING EXERCISE
Out of 73 prefixes, I correctly identified __________.

SUFFIX MATCHING EXERCISE
Out of 29 suffixes, I correctly identified __________.

WHOLE WORD MATCHING EXERCISE
Out of 202 terms, I correctly identified __________.

TRUE/FALSE EXERCISE
Out of 50 true/false questions, I correctly answered __________.

FILL-IN-THE-BLANKS EXERCISE
Out of 65 fill-in-the-blanks questions, I correctly answered __________.

RE-TEST EXERCISE
Out of 202 terms, I correctly identified __________.

Self-Instruction Program

The LEARN-A-TERM program, while designed for use in a classroom situation, is equally well-suited for use by an individual. If you are taking the course independently of an instructor, the following schedule should be used as a guide. While it is important that you follow the prescribed order of study, you may work at your own speed. It is recommended, however, that the various individual sections be completed in one sitting, and that at least a day or two be allowed to elapse before beginning the next section.

PART I — INTRODUCTION AND PRE-TEST

First, read the Introduction to the course on page 1 of the text; then read the Pre-Test Instructions on page 2. Following these instructions, answer the multiple choice questions.

Upon completion of the exercise, record the number of terms you correctly identified in the space provided on page 163.

PART II — WORD/PICTURE ASSOCIATIONS

Referring to the Index of 202 terms, look up the word/picture associations for all those words you did not know on the Pre-Test. Follow the instructions given on page 17.

It will be of additional benefit to you if you write down these word associations as you look them up. Use plain notebook paper; you will not need to keep these sheets—this is primarily a means of reinforcing the memory process.

You may pace yourself in completing this part of the exercise, although it would be desirable to finish looking up all the words and corresponding picture associations in no more than one sitting.

PART III — PREFIX AND SUFFIX MATCHING EXERCISES

Read the instructions for the matching exercises on page 115. Then simply complete the first two exercises and once again refer to the word/picture associations for those suffixes and prefixes you did not know (note that the suffixes and prefixes are grouped in alphabetical order). Once again, write down those associations and definitions for those suffixes and prefixes you did not know.

Record the number of correct answers on both exercises in the space provided on page 163.

PART IV — SUFFIX AND PREFIX CROSSWORD PUZZLES

Read the instructions for the crossword puzzles on page 136. Complete the Suffix Puzzle (page 137) and the Prefix Puzzles (pages 139-141). After checking the solutions in the answer section, again refer to the word/picture associations sections and look up all suffixes and prefixes you did not know.

PART V — WHOLE WORD MATCHING EXERCISE

This exercise is essentially the same as the initial "Pre-Test," although presented in a different format. Once again read the instructions for the matching exercises on page 115. Upon completion of the exercise refer, as before, to the word/picture associations and write out the associations for those words you did not yet know.

Record the number of terms correctly identified in the space provided on page 163.

PART VI — WHOLE WORD CROSSWORD PUZZLES I AND II

Complete Whole Word Crosswords I and II (pages 142-147), and follow the directions as noted above under Part IV.

PART VII — WHOLE WORD CROSSWORD PUZZLE III

Complete Whole Word Crossword III (pages 146-147), once again following the directions as noted under Part IV.

PART VIII — TRUE/FALSE AND FILL-IN-THE-BLANKS EXERCISES

Read the instructions for these exercises on page 125. Then simply answer the questions—as before, refer to the word/picture associations for those words or word-parts missed.

Record the number of questions answered correctly for both exercises in the spaces provided on page 163.

PART IX — RE-TEST

Read the instructions on page 131. This is the same exercise as the initial "Pre-Test," and you should again work at the same speed as you did before.

Record the number of terms correctly identified in the space provided on page 163.

You have now completed the LEARN-A-TERM course in medical terminology. Your score on the Re-Test should show a definite improvement over the score on the initial Pre-Test exercise. There may still be, however, some words you did not get correct. Work on these words independently, using the word/picture memory associations, or any other memory devices you may find helpful, such as creating sentences with these words, or breaking the words down into their various parts and developing new memory associations.

Keep the LEARN-A-TERM text and occasionally refer to it in order to refresh your memory. Hopefully these words and their meanings will stay with you, increasing your understanding and appreciation of your job, and making your working experience more meaningful.

Administration Manual

INTRODUCTION

Learn-A-Term is a modularly designed terminology program for teaching 202 medical terms and 115 medical prefixes and suffixes. These are terms which should be known, understood, and used by competent medical paraprofessionals. The terms taught in this course were selected by medical librarians from several large hospitals and by department chairmen from allied health field schools as being the most important for paraprofessionals in their daily job activities. The methodology for teaching these terms is specifically based on a systems design for education. Performance objectives for each step in the program can be modified, removed, or exchanged with another milestone to provide maximum teaching flexibility and deliver optimum instruction for the student.

Methodology

The overall program performance objective is that a student, upon completion of the program, will use, express correctly, pronounce correctly, and understand 202 medical terms and 115 prefixes and suffixes. The means used for achieving the objective represent a strikingly effective use of modern learning theory. Historically, the use of tests has been to determine the level of *achievement* in a given area by the test taker. It is our contention that tests should only be used as a learning device for both teacher and student. To do so, the use of a test must be to determine the *deficiency* level of a student so that the most effective and fastest devices for filling those deficiencies may be brought to bear. Deficiency levels tell the student what it is that he must learn and at the same time, they tell the teacher what he or she must provide. Tests serve a third major function in the learning process if used appropriately; they can be powerful media for conveying information. We have based the Learn-A-Term teaching methodology on these three principles. This course can be taken individually as a home study course or administered in the classroom in group instruction.

Each step in the program is based on the student's performance in the preceding step. Thus, this program is absolutely and uniquely individualized. Each student sets his own performance objectives depending upon his own needs. For example, in Step I, the student's entry level *deficiency* is diagnosed by the use of a *multiple choice test*. Each of the 202 multiple choice items is keyed to a referent number-letter system. When all of the test items have been answered, and the test corrected, the student goes on to *Step II*. In this step, the student refers to the keyed number-letter system for the items missed. Notice that he is only learning the information for which he has shown a deficiency. Under the number-letter system, the student finds each word divided into root or stem, each term defined, pronunciation for each term, the word used in context, and a mnemonic association for the word. By studying the mnemonic (or writing his own as he is taught to do) the student will more easily remember the word. When he has completed the referrent process for each term he missed, he goes on to *Step III*. In Step III, the student takes a *matching test* on all 202 terms. From the matching test, the student learns which words he still has not learned, the instructor is made aware of the student's learning process, and the conditions for *Step IV* are provided. Using the results of the matching test, the student takes a *fill-in-test* only for the items he missed on the matching test. The purpose of this test is to have the student write out an approximate meaning for the terms he doesn't know. Often, he must look up the word meaning before he can answer the item. When he has completed the fill-in-test, he is given a post-test (multiple choice), on all 202 words.

At each step, the student misses less and less items. Each time he is reinforced for getting other items correct. The retesting of all items serves to backward chain terms he has recently learned. Whereas many students usually miss as many as 75% of the 202 items in Step I, they usually miss less than 5% in Step V, the post-test. At this point, the student begins to work on a series of crossword puzzles using the 202 terms. The puzzles can be given as classroom projects or as homework assignments. At the same time, he is introduced to 69 prefixes and 46 suffixes by use of a matching test. Using the same "test and study" process described above, the student learns the 115 prefixes and suffixes. Crossword exercises are also provided for reinforcing the prefixes and suffixes. The diagram below indicates the decrease in learning deficits evinced by the student as the course proceeds. The individual performance objectives are determined for each new step by the amount the student has learned in the last step. The student learns from each test *what* he doesn't know, and he then studies those terms. He is retested to see what he doesn't know, and he then studies those terms, etc. In each step, he is backward chaining the steps he has just learned at the same time that he is learning new terms.

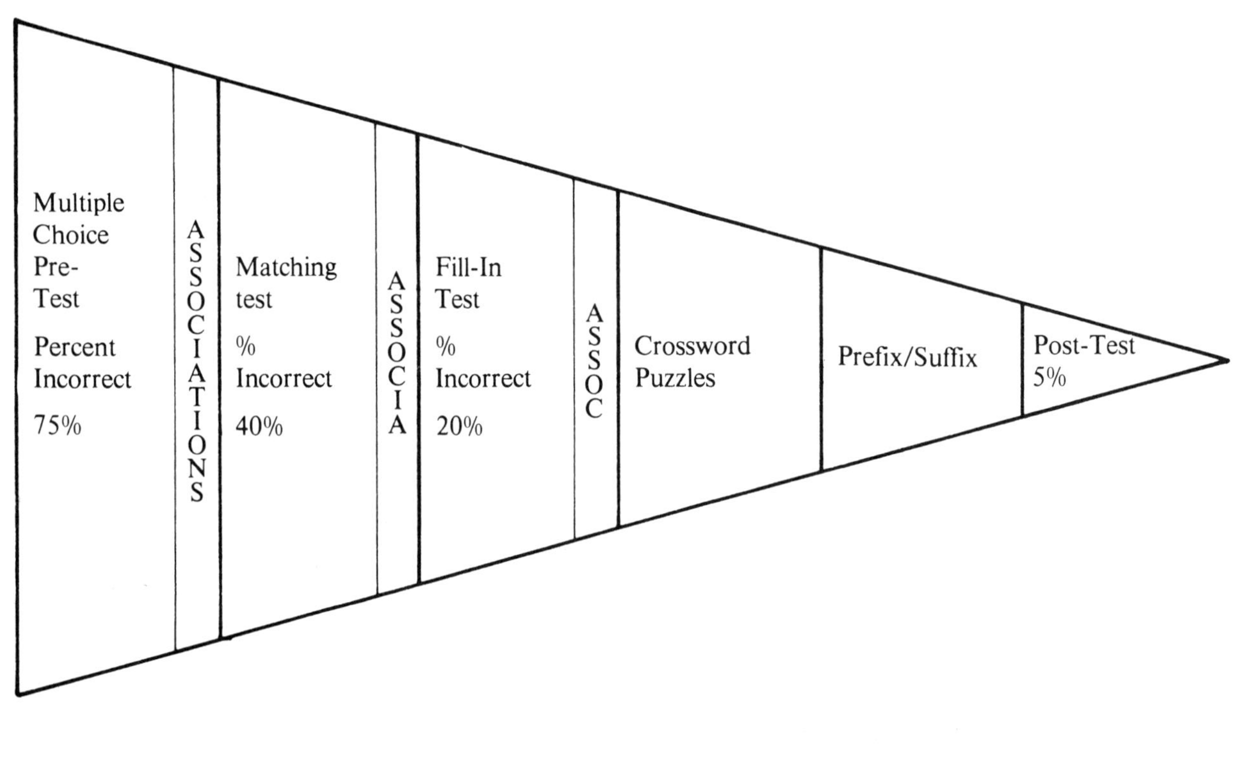

STEPS

I   II   III   IV   V   VI   VII   VIII   IX

% of
Misses

75%   40%   20%   0%   0%   5%